Keto Vegetarian

The Ultimate Guide to the Ketogenic Vegetarian Diet for Permanent Weight Loss and Burn Fat; Includes 90 Easy Low-Carb Plant-Based Recipes and two-week meal plans, Beginner Friendly

By Michelle Thomasson

Table of Contents

Introduction

Chapter 1: What Is The Ketogenic Diet?

Chapter 2: Advantages and Disadvantages of the Keto Diet

Chapter 3: Keto Vegetarian Style

Chapter 4: Shopping For Vegetarian Keto

Chapter 5: Herbs, Spices, and Sauces

Chapter 6: Breakfast Recipes

1. Curried Tofu Scramble
2. Maple Oatmeal
3. Scrambled Eggs with Cheese
4. Egg Breakfast Muffins
5. Tomato Omelet
6. Mediterranean Breakfast Burrito
7. Banana Pancakes
8. Chia Breakfast Pudding
9. Five Ingredient Baked Pancake
10. Baked Eggs with Tomato and Spinach
11. Peppers and Onions Scrambled Eggs
12. Avocado and Poached Egg
13. Spinach Mozzarella Frittata
14. Baked Italian Skillet Eggs
15. Huevos Rancheros

16. Baked Avocado Eggs

17. Sweet Potato Hash Egg Muffin

18. Baked Scrambled Eggs

19. Vegetable Quiche

20. Egg Drop Soup

21. Mushroom Sandwich with Eggs and Greens

22. Punjabi Egg Curry

23. Eggs with Brussel Sprouts

24. Cinnamon Custard

25. Cream Cheese Pancakes

Chapter 7: Lunch and Dinner Recipes

1. Cauliflower Rice and Mushroom Risotto

2. Grilled Eggplant Roll-Ups

3. Eggplant Gratin with Feta Cheese

4. Stuffed Zucchini with Marinara and Goat Cheese

5. Herb and Halloumi Tomato Salad

6. Greek Fattoush Salad

7. Veggie Stuffed Peppers

8. Eggplant Chickpea Stew

9. Springtime Greek Soup

10. Spicy Lentil Soup*

11. Tomato and Red Pepper Soup

12. Zucchini Soup

13. Tuscany Vegetable Soup

14. Cheddar Cheese and Roast Cauliflower Soup

15. Cabbage Soup

16. Nicoise Salad

17. Sprout Wraps

18. Cheesy Gratin Zucchini

19. Cilantro Lime Coleslaw

20. Caprese Tomatoes with Basil Dressing

21. Greek Collard wraps

22. Zucchini and Spinach Lasagna

23. Fried Goat Cheese with Charred Veggies

24. Vegetarian Club Salad

25. Spiral Zucchini and Grape Tomatoes

26. Cauliflower Fried Rice

27. Cheesy Broccoli and Cauliflower Rice

28. Mediterranean Pasta

29. Roast Baby Eggplant

30. Squash and Sweet Potato Patties

31. Chickpea Salad

32. Greek Spaghetti Squash

33. Tomato, Squash, and Red Pepper Gratin

34. Cheesy Cauliflower Soup

35. Stuffed Artichokes

36. Lima Bean Casserole

37. Kale and Chickpea Salad with Poppy seed Lemon Dressing

38. Eggplant Casserole

39. Butternut Squash with Mustard Vinaigrette

40. Corn and Okra Casserole

Chapter 8: Keto Sauces

1. Avocado Cilantro Sauce

2. Pesto Sauce

3. Mustard Sauce

4. Lemon Herb Sauce

5. Creamy Alfredo

6. Marinara Sauce

7. White Cheese Sauce

8. Sweet Soy Sauce

9. Pepper Sauce

10. Whole Egg Mayonnaise

11. Guacamole

12. Avocado Garlic Caesar Dressing

13. Lemon Curd

14. Ranch Dressing

15. Italian Dressing

Chapter 9: Keto Desserts

1. Cheesecake Keto Fat Bombs

2. Cinnamon Sugar Donuts

3. One Minute Brownie

4. Peanut Butter Balls

5. Cinnamon Roll Cheesecake

6. Brownies

7. No Churn Ice Cream

8. White Chocolate Peanut Butter Blondies

9. Chocolate Chip Cookies

10. Chocolate Frosty

Chapter 10: Two Week Meal Plan

Chapter 11: Making the Keto Diet Your Own

Chapter 12: Living Keto In The Real World

Conclusion

Introduction

Anyone who makes a conscious decision to eat better and be healthier should be applauded. After all, it is not an easy thing in the world we live in today to always make the choices that are the best for our bodies when we are making food choices. There are tempting food choices on every corner. Some blocks contain five separate drives thus that are there just to tempt you with their offerings.

But you have made the decision not only to live a vegetarian lifestyle but also to live a keto lifestyle. This should get you double reward points because you have not only chosen two of the diets most guaranteed to give the results you want but also two of the diet that is guaranteed to make people look at you and scratch their heads in confusion.

Being a vegetarian in a world full of meat eaters is not an easy task. And now you want to be able to take advantage of the benefits that a ketogenic diet will give to you. You want to be able to double your weight loss efforts without doing a lot of extra work. And this is the book that you need to get you started and keep you on the right track. Because this book, *Keto Vegetarian Diet: The Ultimate Guide to the Ketogenic Vegetarian Diet for Permanent Weight Loss and Burn Fat; Includes Easy Low-Carb*

Plant-Based Recipes, Beginner Friendly by Michelle Cole is the definitive book that will help you reach all of the goals that you want to reach.

See, vegetarianism is not so much a diet as it is a way to live your life. It is a lifestyle choice. So is living the keto life. Keto is not a diet plan although it is often referred to as one. Rather keto is a way of life, a totally new lifestyle that you will be able to adapt by making just a few little changes to your everyday eating habits. And this book is the book that will give you all the information that you need so that you, too, can be successful in your new lifestyle journey.

In this book, you will learn a little bit about the history of the keto diet. See, the keto diet has been around for a lot longer than most people think it has. And it was originally used for purposes other than just weight loss. The weight loss aspect of keto living has been a recent development and pursuit and this book will explain exactly how to achieve that goal. By understanding where keto came from and all of the ways, it can be used you will have the power to be able to make the most intelligent choices about your life with keto.

You will learn which foods will be your new best friends and which foods you will need to learn to live without. The eating plan may seem a bit restrictive in the beginning but you will soon become accustomed to the restrictions and they will no longer seem so restrictive. You will find that the choices available to you on the keto diet plan are much more open and friendly than you probably thought they were.

You will find keto friendly menu options for breakfast, lunch, and dinner. You will learn which herbs and spices will make your dishes taste more appetizing. You will see how to balance your intake of fats, proteins, and carbs in order to create the perfect keto meal plans.

This book contains recipes for many wonderful meal options. You will learn ways to use vegetables that you may never have thought of before. But the recipes in this book are easy to follow and some even have pictures so that you will know exactly what this particular dish is supposed to look like when you set the finished product on the table. And these recipes are suitable for any member of the family, so there is no need to make differently dished to accommodate different tastes. Everyone in the family can eat these foods and they will be healthier if they do so.

There is even a section for keto friendly desserts because what would like to be without the occasional cookie or piece of fudge to sweeten the deal? Living a vegetarian keto lifestyle does not mean giving up everything yummy, and this is the book that will prove that to you.

Chapter 1: What Is The Ketogenic Diet?

In one form or another ketogenic, or keto, the diet has been in use for centuries. In ancient Greece, physicians treated various diseases, especially the disease of epilepsy, by making changes in their patient's diets. Many Greek physicians believed that there was a physical and rational basis to use dietary therapy to cure illnesses and conditions.

The first study of a modern type was not conducted until the twentieth century. A group of patients with epilepsy was treated with a vegetarian diet that was low in calories. Those who maintained strict adherence to the diet were able to greatly decrease or end their seizures. Scientists who studied the results of this experiment found that there were three compounds that are water soluble and are located in the liver of healthy people who were adhering to a very low calorie or a starvation diet. They coined the term 'ketone bodies' as a name to call these compounds. Other doctors built on this research and discovered that the body could be made to produce ketone bodies when it was fed a high fat low carbohydrate diet. Because of the ketone bodies, the term 'ketogenic' was first used.

The first keto diets varied widely in the ratio of fats to proteins consumed until a pediatrician tried using the diet on his patients to see if it could reduce or eliminate their symptoms of epilepsy. His formula was for the patient to consume only one gram of protein for every pound of body weight, fifteen to twenty grams of carbs per day, and the rest of the caloric intake would be made up of fat. Besides reducing the seizures of epilepsy doctors noted that their patients slept longer and more soundly, had an improved level of alertness, and experienced better overall behavior with very few or no side effects.

The keto diet was widely used as a treatment for epilepsy until the middle to the latter part of the twentieth century when anti-convulsing drugs became more readily available and highly popular. Taking a pill is much easier than sticking to a rigid diet. So the keto diet fell out of favor until the 1990s, when a television producer and his wife were searching for a treatment for their young son, who suffered from debilitating seizures that even high doses of medicine did not stop. Their child did so well on the keto diet that they promoted it to everyone who would listen, and the diet was once again popular.

In normal physical processes, the human body will burn carbs for energy. The body turns carbs into sugar, or glucose, during the process of digestion.

When people eat the pancreas gets a signal from the brain to produce insulin to help take the sugar produced by digestion through the bloodstream and into the cells. The insulin is actually the key that gets the blood sugar into the cells. The pancreas will produce as much insulin as the body needs to transport and disperse the amount of blood sugar the body has to get rid of. The body will also store a precise amount of blood sugar in the liver in the form of glycogen. This is a type of emergency store in case the body faces starvation before the next meal appears.

The problem begins when there is too much blood sugar, as usually happens when people eat a high sugar high carb diet. Eventually, the cells will have all of the glucose that they need and they will begin to ignore the insulin when it comes knocking on the cell door. This is known as insulin resistance. The body then needs to find a place to put all of this excess glucose so it stores it as fat beginning around the organs of the abdomen and then spreading out to other areas of the body.

The predominant goal when following the keto diet is to lower the consumption of carbs enough to burn body fat enough to cause massive weight loss. The other part of that goal is to feel fewer food cravings, especially for sugary foods, while making the body feel full with less food consumed.

When the consumption of carbs is restricted to a low level the body needs to find a new source of energy for the cells to be able to function. The body will first begin to burn the glycogen that is stored in the liver when the supply of blood sugar in the bloodstream decreases. The liver can store enough glycogen to fuel the body for about forty-eight hours. After that time the body will search for other ways to obtain fuel for the body to use. The liver will use the stored fat in the body to break it down to make fuel.

Your body goes through a perfectly normal metabolic process called ketosis when it begins to burn stored fat for fuel. This is a perfectly normal process the body goes through when access to carbs is limited or eliminated. The body produces ketones when it goes into ketosis and this is what the body uses for fuel instead of carbs. This is a feature that was built into the body ages ago to keep early man from starving to death during times when food was not readily available.

Ketosis is the name given to the body's function of making ketones from stored fat for fuel for the body. The body will usually enter ketosis after about three or four days of eating a low carb diet. The main purpose of following the keto diet is to get the body to enter ketosis because this means the body has begun burning stored fat. Most people enter ketosis with few to no symptoms, and some people experience what is called the 'keto flu' because the symptoms feel much like having the flu.

During the beginning of ketosis, the person may experience very bad breath. This happens because the body is breaking down toxins with the breakdown of stored fat, and toxins are removed from the body in three ways—through urination, through sweating, and through the respiratory system. So your body is sending out toxins with every exhale. This symptom will only last a few days, and more tooth brushing or use of mouthwash will help lessen the symptoms.

Also when going into ketosis you will probably feel less hungry. This is because the body is learning to use food more efficiently. This is also because carbs are digested quickly and leave you feeling hungry soon after eating them. And protein and fat take longer to digest, so you will feel less hungry than before.

The keto flu, like the flu that is brought on by a virus, can leave you feeling exhausted. Part of this is due to the decreased intake of carbs that give instant energy to the body. Part of this may be caused by slight dehydration.

Excess fat stored in the body holds water, which is why the first few pounds lost on any diet are water weight. You can combat this fatigue by drinking more water and by drinking sugar-free sports drinks with electrolytes.

And during the first few days of ketosis, you will likely see a decrease in your performance while exercising. While exercise is important to weight loss it might be necessary during this time to lessen the intensity of your workouts. Also, your muscles need time to become adjusted to the difference in the source of the fuel they are receiving.

Some people experience issues with the digestive system like diarrhea or constipation. Constipation is usually more of an issue that diarrhea is. Diarrhea comes from an increased intake of fat in the diet and your body will become used to the increase of fat in your diet. Constipation comes from not drinking enough water and from not eating enough vegetables. There are certain low carb veggies that are allowed on the keto diet and these should be eaten daily to keep your system regular.

Following a ketogenic plan should not be thought of as a diet plan but it should be viewed as a lifestyle change. This is a way of eating that can be done for many years. As long as you follow the keto diet you will continue to enjoy the benefits of the keto diet.

Chapter 2: Advantages and Disadvantages of the Keto Diet

Every new diet or lifestyle change has its own set of advantages and disadvantages. But the advantages of the keto diet far outweigh the disadvantages for most people, which is why more people begin following the keto diet all the time.

One definite advantage of the keto diet is lowered insulin production. Whenever you eat the brain signals the pancreas to make more insulin. The insulin is what makes the energy around to the cells. If you eat too much food then the body will make too much insulin. Eventually, the cells will stop responding to the insulin and this is called insulin resistance. When insulin resistance happens and there is more blood sugar than the cells of the body need, then it is stored in and around the abdomen. This is known as a metabolic disease. When the stored fat is consumed for energy the body will only make the amount of insulin it really needs and the abdominal fat will decrease, thus eliminating metabolic syndrome.

Metabolic syndrome might be one of the factors in the development of Type 2 Diabetes. This type of diabetes is caused by poor lifestyle choices such as obesity. When less food is consumed then the level of blood sugar decreases and high blood sugar is one of the markers of diabetes. Following a keto diet will help control the levels of sugar in the blood and, in turn, diseases and conditions caused by high blood sugar.

A keto diet might also be beneficial for people who have Parkinson's disease or Alzheimer's disease. When the body gets fuel from ketones instead of carbs the brain must also use these ketones to fuel its processes. There is evidence that using ketones for brain fuel decreases cognitive issues in people with Alzheimer's disease and balance issues in people who have Parkinson's disease. Some studies show that people who have been diagnosed as bipolar will suffer fewer mood swings when following a keto diet.

And while following a keto diet will not cure or prevent cancer it is certainly a helpful addition to regular cancer treatments. Cancer cells can't use ketones for food the way they can use glucose, so they eventually starve to death on a keto diet. And the keto diet can help women with Polycystic Ovary Disease because one of the main causes of that disease is obesity.

Perhaps the biggest benefit to the body is the good effects a keto diet can have on the cardiovascular system. Heart disease and high blood are directly caused by obesity, as is a hardening of the arteries. The bodies of overweight people make more arteries and veins in order to feed the larger body size, and this causes the heart to work harder as it struggles to pump blood throughout the body. And excess fat can cause the arteries to harden because little clumps of fat can break loose and get caught on the insides of arteries whose walls have been stretched thin by high blood pressure. When these clumps gather they cause a blockage in the artery.

Your joints will feel better with every pound you lose. Every pound of excess weight on the body causes four pounds of pressure on the knees. So losing excess weight lessens the strain on the joints in the lower body. It will also lessen the amount of inflammation in the body. When muscles and joints feel strain they release chemicals that the body treats like an infection that needs to be eliminated, so it sends white blood cells to combat the inflammation, which causes more inflammation.

Like every other diet plan, the keto diet does have some disadvantages. The drawbacks are not as severe as the ones associated with some diets, but they should be considered before beginning the diet.

The keto diet will take some getting used to. Getting your body fully adapted to the keto diet can take a week or two and some people are very uncomfortable during this time period. This is when the symptoms of keto flu hit and the body may become dehydrated. Both of these conditions will pass eventually.

The dramatic increase in the intake of fat can cause stomach issues for some people. Diarrhea and constipation are common, but both of those can easily be overcome by adding fluids to the diet, particularly fluids that contain electrolytes. And there might be some bouts of nausea during this time because the body needs time for the liver, pancreas, and gall bladder to adjust to the change in food intake.

Certain food groups are suddenly off limits. Carbs are heavily restricted, and there is no room in the keto diet for grains and certain vegetables. And the foods that are allowed will require extra preparation if you intend to be successful at the diet. This will be especially important to you if you want to cook several days' worth of meals at once or prepare a dinner large enough to leave some leftover for tomorrow's lunch. And some people struggle with social gatherings, particularly those that revolve around food. You might struggle to find appropriate menu items at functions like these.

Not everyone is an appropriate candidate for following the keto diet. Children certainly should not restrict carbs to the level called for by the keto diet because they are still growing and need all the nutrition they can consume. Ketosis might have harmful effects on the fetus, so pregnant women should not attempt a low carb diet. Also, women who are nursing may find that the keto diet does not give them enough carbs to make a good supply of healthy milk for the baby. People who have Type 2 Diabetes and take insulin replacement hormones should proceed cautiously, since their medication and ketosis may not be a good mix. Anyone who suffers from gall bladder disease or has had their gall bladder removed may find the increased level of fat difficult to digest, at least in the beginning. And people who have kidney stones will need to take special care to remain well-hydrated while on the diet.

Overall the benefits of following the keto diet far outweigh any negatives you might run into. The opportunity to be healthier for the rest of your life is certainly worth a few days of fatigue and more time spent on getting your meal ready. By following a meal plan that is rich in nutrition without all the bad foods you will achieve this goal of a healthier lifestyle.

Chapter 3: Keto Vegetarian Style

Given that meat is one of the cornerstones of the keto diet the vegetarian community has long been thought to have been unable to take full advantage of the keto lifestyle. But keto is no longer off limits for the population that follows a vegetarian diet. Many people have been able to rearrange the diet plan to make it work for those people who do not eat meat.

Following the keto diet requires you to limit carbs in favor of eating protein and fats. In fact, fats make up the bulk of the calories consumed daily. Doing the diet as a vegetarian has its own set of challenges that are unique in the world of keto. It might require a little bit of extra effort to make sure you get the right amount of protein in your diet, but the diet is completely accessible to everyone no matter what their dietary style is.

Following a keto diet that is heavily plant-based give you the benefits of eating a diet that is high in fat without eating meats which can sometimes lead to inflammation in the body. Also, eating a keto diet based on plant nutrition gives the same health benefits as a keto diet based on meat protein. The key is to make sure you get enough healthy fats in your daily diet. High-fat vegetarian foods are readily available in the right sources.

Many vegetarians rely on grains and pasta to fill up the empty spaces on their plates and this may make the first few days on the keto diet especially difficult for them since these foods are not allowed when following the keto diet. There are plenty of healthy carbs that will help to round out your meal and will give you all the ketogenic benefits a meat-based keto diet plan.

You will want to invest in a good multivitamin and remember to take it daily. People who follow a vegetarian diet may already be at risk of not getting enough omega 3 fatty acids, calcium, iron, zinc, vitamin D, and vitamin B-12. Following the keto diet will make food choices even more restrictive. For example, grains that would provide a source of vitamin B-12 are not allowed on the keto diet. And you will need to take special care to get the right amount of proteins in your diet since these are especially important for your skin, muscles, and bones.

Following a vegetarian diet is one of the healthiest ways to live and one of the best methods available for sustained weight loss. Maximizing weight loss is the ultimate goal of the keto diet. It is quite possible for a vegetarian to be overweight, unfortunately. Most vegetarian diets are low in fat and overloaded in carbohydrates. Consuming too many sugars and carbs will lead to gaining weight. So if the typical diet of most vegetarians is not helping you with its emphasis on a lowered fat intake and a higher carbohydrate intake, then the vegetarian keto diet is the right one for you. It restricts the intake of carbohydrates while promoting the consumption of the proteins and fats that the body needs to maintain good health.

The body will eventually enter a state of ketosis whenever carb intake is limited, whether a person does or does not eat products that come from animals. The state of ketosis will promote a reduction of weight because it will naturally suppress the hormones that let you know that you are hungry, so your appetite will decrease.

When following a keto vegetarian meal plan it is necessary to put your focus on natural whole foods. These foods will help you get all the nutrients you need every day and will also provide plenty of low carb options that digest slowly and keep you feeling fuller longer. This will also help you to maintain higher energy levels throughout the day. Avoid processed foods and refined foods that will not benefit your body in any way.

So where do the necessary fats and proteins come from on a vegetarian keto diet if they are not coming from the consumption of meat? You will get your fats and proteins from eggs and dairy products, with a few nuts thrown in to make everything interesting. Dairy products, especially, are a great addition to the vegetarian diet in order to maintain needed levels of fats and proteins in your diet. When you are looking for options in the dairy department look for those that are low in carbohydrates and do not have any added sugars or flavorings (flavorings are often made from sugar even if they don't say so). Butter and ghee will be your new best friends.

Any vegetarian who wants to eat clean and cut out carbs should follow the keto diet plan. Make a strong commitment that you will eat a wide variety of foods that are approved and your new diet path will be smooth.

Chapter 4: Shopping For Vegetarian Keto

A keto vegetarian diet deftly joins the keto lifestyle with vegetarianism. Eating a vegetarian diet means typically that you do not eat poultry, fish, or beef—or any other meat, and there are different variations that depend on the individual and their food preferences. A keto vegetarian diet will feature foods that are not meat and will feature foods that are high in fat and low in carbs.

Even though carbs are restricted on the keto diet there are plenty of good carb options available and some should be eaten daily. Remember this diet is low carb, not no-carb. There are a good number of good tasting carbohydrates that you will be allowed to eat on this diet. The key will be getting enough protein in your daily diet.

You may see opinions about the keto diet that say that all foods must be in the purest form possible. Some people think that eggs should only come from chickens that have been fed an all-natural organic diet and dairy products should only come from cows that are free roaming or fed an organic diet. All vegetables and fruits must be organic. While eating food in its purest form is desirable and would certainly be good for your body, it is not always possible or even necessary. The first consideration is usually money because these types of foods are more expensive than regular foods in the same category. If you are living in the country it may be difficult to locate organic foods. And even though big box stores and chain stores are coming around to the organic style, it can be difficult finding organic foods at a price you can afford. It is nothing to worry about because as long as you follow the guidelines of the diet you will lose weight and eat quite well.

Beginning in the dairy case you will find the largest source of the protein for your new diet plan. Remember that cheese will have some carbs but they will be a minimal amount. You will need to get ghee and butter because these will be good sources of fats. Ghee is nothing more than butter that has been heated to clarify it by removing the water and the milk solids. You will want to buy heavy cream to use in recipes and as a whipped topping for a bowl of berries for dessert. Hard cheeses are better than soft cheeses, and cheese that is already shredded will have a slightly higher carb count because of the milk that is used to make them easy to shred.

For a one ounce serving the following cheeses have these amounts of protein and carbs:

Cheese	Net Carbs	Protein
Swiss cheese	1.51 grams net carbs	8 grams protein
Romano cheese	1.03 grams net carbs	9 grams protein
Ricotta cheese	.86 grams net carbs	3.5 grams protein
Provolone cheese	.60 grams net carbs	7.3 grams protein
Pepper Jack	.5 grams net carbs	6.8 grams protein

Parmesan cheese	.91 grams net carbs	12 grams protein
Neufchatel cheese	.83 grams net carbs	2.6 grams protein
Muenster cheese	.31 grams net carbs	6.9 grams protein
Mozzarella cheese	.79 grams net carbs	6.9 grams protein
Monterey cheese	.19 grams net carbs	4 Grams protein
Jarlsberg	.5 grams net carbs	6 grams protein
Halloumi	.6 grams net carb	6.3 grams protein
Havarti cheese	.79 grams net carbs	4 Grams protein
Gruyere cheese	.10 grams net carbs	8.5 grams protein
Gouda cheese	.63 grams net carbs	7.1 grams protein
Gorgonzola	.66 grams net carbs	6 grams protein
Feta cheese	1.16 grams net carb	4 grams protein
Edam cheese	.4 grams net carbs	7.1 grams protein
Cream cheese	.75 grams net carbs	2.14 grams protein
Cottage cheese	.76 grams net carbs	3.5 grams protein
Colby cheese	.72 grams net carbs	6.7 grams protein
Cheddar cheese	.36 grams net carbs	7 grams protein
Camembert cheese	.13 grams net carbs	6 grams protein
Brie cheese	.13 grams net carbs	5.9 grams protein
Blue cheese	.66 grams net carbs	6.1 grams protein
Asiago	.91 grams net carbs	10.14 grams protein
American cheese	1.97 grams net carbs	5 grams protein

When you are counting your carbohydrates remember to count only net carbs. Net carbs are determined by taking the total carb count and subtracting the amount of dietary fiber in the item.

Dietary fiber is also a carb but the body cannot digest it, and fiber passes straight through the body and is eliminated as waste. So the amount leftover is the net carb count for that food item.

Also in the dairy case, you will find the following items with these nutritional counts per one ounce:

Butter
.01 grams net carbs   .24 grams protein   4 grams fat

Ghee
0 grams net carbs   0 grams protein   14 grams fat

Greek Yogurt
1 grams net carbs   2.8 grams protein   3 grams fat

Heavy cream
.83 grams net carbs   .61 grams protein   11 grams fat

Sour cream
1.21 grams net carbs   .9 grams protein   6 grams fat

Eggs
.6 grams net carbs   6 grams protein   5 grams fat

The first five items will be used to flavor your food and as a good source of the fat, you will need to consume daily. Eggs will be a major source of protein while you are on the keto diet. Make sure to buy Greek yogurt and not the plain yogurt; it has more protein and fewer carbs than regular yogurt does. Yogurt does not have high-fat content but it is good to have on hand for a quick snack when needed. When you are buying oil to use any oil is carb free and high in fat and do not overlook lard just because it has been around forever.

In the center of the store there are vegetarian choices that will enhance your daily diet and are low in the carb or have no carbs that you should include in your daily dietary choices:

Club soda, tea, and coffee
Hot sauce*
Mayonnaise, full fat*
Mustard*
Olives*
Sauerkraut
Sugar-free sports drinks
Vegetable Broth
Vinegar

*Check the food label for any added starches or sugars

The produce counter is where you will need to be more careful of your choices, and it is also where the bulk of your food choices will come from. Vegetables and fruits have carbs. Some veggies and fruits have fewer carbs than others and are allowed almost freely on the keto diet. Other fruits and veggies have higher amounts of carbs and will not be eaten as often.

These are the best vegetables with the lowest carb count for a three-ounce serving:

Artichoke	3 grams net carbs
Arugula	.5 grams net carbs
Asparagus	2 grams net carbs
Avocado	2 grams net carbs
Bean sprouts	.4 grams net carbs
Bok choy	1 gram net carbs
Broccoli	4 grams net carbs
Brussel sprouts	5 grams net carbs
Cabbage	3 grams net carbs
Cauliflower	3 grams net carbs
Celery	2.4 grams net carbs
Collard greens	1 gram net carbs
Cucumber	3 grams net carbs
Eggplant	3 grams net carbs
Green beans	4 grams net carbs
Green bell peppers	3 grams net carbs
Kale	3 grams net carbs
Lettuce (all types)	2 grams net carbs
Mushrooms	2 grams net carbs
Mustard greens	1.5 grams net carbs
Okra	3 grams net carbs
Radishes	1 gram net carbs
Red bell peppers	4 grams net carbs

Red cabbage	3 grams net carbs
Shallots	3 grams net carbs
Spaghetti squash	3 grams net carbs
Spinach	1 gram net carbs
Tomato	3 grams net carbs
Turnip	4 grams net carbs
Yellow bell peppers	5 grams net carbs
Zucchini	3 grams net carbs

Your body will need some carbs every day and these vegetables are low in net carbs and will provide good sources of fiber and will allow you to eat a bit more if you feel the need on certain days. There are vegetables that can be eaten occasionally that are higher in net carbs but still have a place in the keto vegetarian diet:

Beets	7 grams net carbs
Carrot	7 grams net carbs
Corn	16 grams net carbs
Edamame (soybeans)	7 grams net carbs
Onion	8 grams net carbs
Parsnips	13 grams net carbs
Peas	9 grams net carbs
Potato	15 grams net carbs

Rutabaga	6 grams net carbs
Sweet potatoes	17 grams net carbs

The fruit counter is where you will need to be really careful. Most fruits are medium to high on the level of carbs and should be enjoyed only sometimes. There are a few fruits that weigh in low on the carbohydrate scale and these counts are for a three-ounce serving:

Blackberries	4 grams net carbs
Blackberries	5 grams net carbs
Cantaloupe	7 grams net carbs
Coconut (meat)	6 grams net carbs
Lemon	6 grams net carbs
Lime	6 grams net carbs
Pumpkin	4 grams net carbs
Raspberries	5 grams net carbs
Strawberries	6 grams net carbs
Watermelon	7 grams net carbs

Other fruits are higher on the carbohydrate scale. Remember the carb count has to do with the sugar count and these fruits contain more fruit sugar than the ones in the previous list. This does not mean they should be ignored but that they should not be a regular part of your diet:

Apple	12 grams net carbs
Banana	20 grams net carbs
Cherries	10 grams net carbs
Clementine	10 grams net carbs
Grapes	16 grams net carbs
Kiwi	12 grams net carbs
Mango	13 grams net carbs
Orange	9 grams net carbs
Peach	8 grams net carbs
Pear	12 grams net carbs
Pineapple	12 grams net carbs
Plum	10 grams net carbs

The fruit is not necessary for a healthy diet. Any nutrients that you can get from the fruit you can get from vegetables. Fruit is just a nice addition to the daily diet and it can take the place of the pies and donuts you will no longer be eating. The key to eating fruit on the keto diet is to do it in moderation.

Also to be eaten in moderation are the following foods. They can still be a part of your diet because they provide needed nutrients, but for the serving size they carry a large number of carbs per one ounce serving:

Almonds	6 grams net carbs	6 grams protein
Cashews	9 grams net carbs	5 grams protein
Hazelnuts	4.7 grams net carbs	4.2 grams protein
Macadamia nuts	3.9 grams net carbs	2.2 grams protein

Peanuts	4.6 grams net carbs	7 grams protein
Pistachios	8 grams net cars	6 grams protein
Walnuts	3.9 grams net carbs	4.3 grams protein

When planning your keto vegetarian diet you need to decide first how low you will go with your carb count. Although some die-hard keto activists say you must go no higher than twenty grams of net carbs per day that really is not true. If you are going strict keto, the plan that will almost guarantee that you go into ketosis almost immediately, then you should keep your net carb count below twenty grams per day. However, there is also the low-carb diet which allows you to eat up to fifty grams of net carbs each day, and the moderate carb diet which allows you to eat up to one hundred grams of net carbs each day. Following the strict twenty-gram keto plan is what many people think of when they think of eliminating carbs from the diet. But on a vegetarian plan, it might not be possible to go that low and still get enough nutrition. Also, different people gain and lose weight in different ways, and some people will enter a state of ketosis on one of the higher carb plans. So choose the plan that best fits your lifestyle and your needs. It is always possible, to begin with, a moderate carb diet and work your way down if true keto is your goal.

Do not overlook the freezer section when grocery shopping. Vegetables and fruits that are frozen are just as healthy as fresh ones and sometimes even healthier. And do not buy foods that you know you will not eat. Mushrooms are great on a low carb diet but if you absolutely cannot stand the taste or texture then there is no sense in buying them.

And don't be afraid to be a bit creative here. After all, this is your menu and the food you will eat. Check out different recipes and make changes. You might find a recipe that calls for collard greens but you prefer the taste of mustard greens. Go ahead and substitute! As long as you consume the proper amounts of nutrients for your body and your lifestyle while monitoring your carb intake, then anything is possible. You definitely will be surprised at how amazingly flexible this eating style really is.

Chapter 5: Herbs, Spices, and Sauces

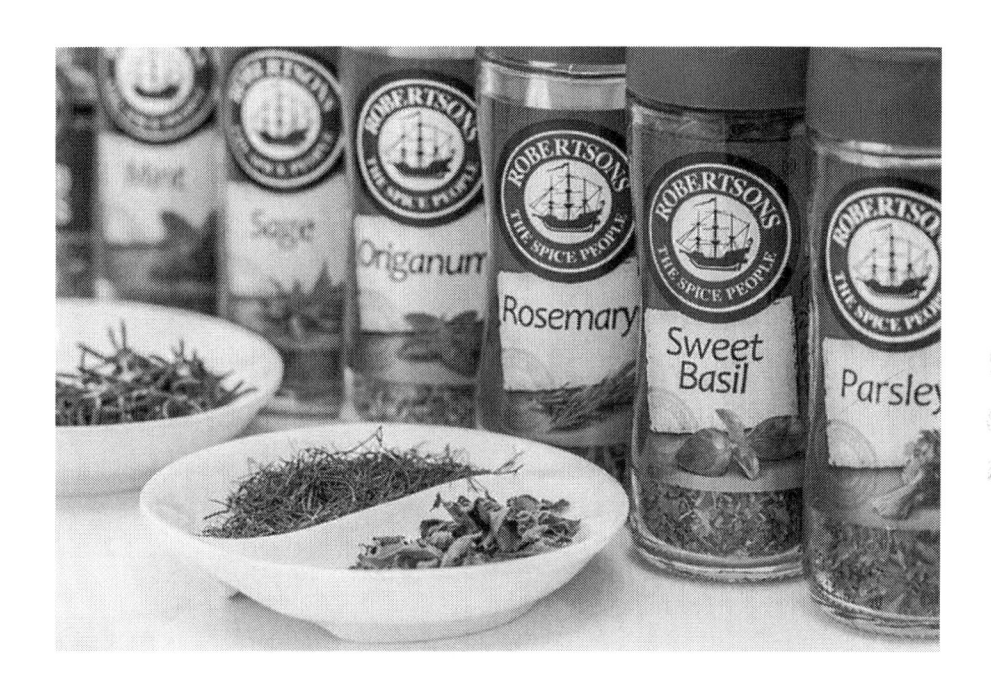

When you make the switch to a lower carb diet you will find yourself reading food labels in search of hidden starches and sugars that could completely derail any progress you have made. But you also do not want to eat bland tasteless food. But when you begin your journey and start reading all those little labels you may be shocked at how many seasonings, sauces, and spice mixes are full of added carbohydrates disguised as anti-caking agents, fillers, sugars, and whatever else the manufacturer decides to put into them. These additives are not necessarily bad because they are edible; they are just not necessarily good for you and the new lifestyle you are following.

There are a number of ways to season and flavor the food you will eat on the keto vegetarian diet. Since you are not eating meat you will not have the advantage of the flavor that comes naturally from meat fat, so you will need to make the flavor up in other ways. And this means becoming familiar with, and using, keto friendly sauces, herbs, and spice.

The following spices and herbs have less than one gram of net carbs per each tablespoon:

Basil – mild to medium flavor good when used in tomato sauces or pesto or sprinkled on top of salads
Black pepper – can be used on any food you want to put it on

Chinese 5-spice – a blend of peppercorns, anise, fennel seed, cloves, and cinnamon this spice adds a bold flavor to green beans, broccoli, asparagus, and any dish with a decided Asian flavor

Cinnamon powder – a mellow spice that goes with many fruits and vegetables like apples, pumpkin, squash, and yogurt

Cloves – a strong spice used with pumpkin, apples, and any type of mixed vegetable dish or vegetable soup

Coriander – since coriander is often used in Indian and Mexican dishes it goes well with potatoes, tomatoes, bell peppers, and onions as well as in sauces and soups

Garam masala – a warm seasoning made of peppercorns, nutmeg, coriander, cumin, cloves, cardamom, and cinnamon and adds depth and warmth to any soup and is traditionally used in Indian cuisine

Ginger powder – ginger is a light spice that goes well with almost any food, particularly foods with an Asian twist. It is also used in making fruit and veggie smoothies

Mint – strong flavor good when used in tomatoes, spinach, potatoes, peas, green beans, cucumber, corn, celery, and carrots as well as tomato and pea soups

Tarragon – subtle flavor good when used in carrots, asparagus, artichokes, fava beans, and eggs

These herbs and spices have less than six grams of carbs in each tablespoon:

Cayenne (3 grams) – an especially hot form of pepper that should be used sparingly but should be used in any dish where you would like a little kick

Chili powder (4.1 grams) – a mix of paprika, oregano, garlic powder, cumin, and cayenne that can also be used in almost any dish

Curry powder (3.7 grams) – a mix of ginger, cardamom, white pepper, coriander, turmeric, and dried yellow mustard it is widely used in Indian cuisine and especially for soups and sauces

Garlic powder (6 grams) – can be used in any dish where you would like the flavor of garlic without the chunks of a clove of garlic

Ground cumin (2.75 grams) – Works well in any vegetable dish or soup recipe

Onion powder (5.4 grams) – this is used for any dish where you would like the flavor of onion without the onion chunks

Oregano (3.3 grams) – a strong herb best used in soups and sauces

Paprika (3.8 grams) – a subtle herb that goes well with cheese dishes, onions, and almost any salad or veggie medley, mostly used for color but does have a milk flavor

Pumpkin pie spice (3.9 grams) – used for flavoring pumpkin for pie filling

Turmeric powder (4.4 grams) – a staple in Indian dishes it also goes well with sautéed vegetables or spaghetti squash

Vinegar can also be used to add flavor to vegetable dishes but be very careful when using balsamic vinegar since it is loaded with extra sugar.

Here are some popular types of vinegar and their carb counts for one tablespoon:

Less than three grams	Less than one gram
Balsamic vinegar (2.7 grams)	Apple cider vinegar
Soy sauce (1.2 grams)	Distilled vinegar
Tamari soy sauce (1 gram)	Red wine vinegar
	White wine vinegar

Red wine vinegar and white wine vinegar do have a tiny trace of alcohol. They are made by allowing diluted wine to ferment. Any alcohol content will be burned off during cooking processes.

And fresh herbs, when used properly, will add a distinct flavor and taste to any dish you create. The following fresh herbs have less than one gram of carbs in each tablespoon:

Basil	Oregano
Bay leaf	Parsley
Cilantro	Rosemary
Dill	Sage
Jalapeno	Spearmint
Lavender	Thyme
Lemongrass	

Many of these fresh herbs are used as a garnish for smoothies or ground up to sprinkle over salads. By using herbs and spices whenever possible your food will not be dull and boring.

Chapter 6: Breakfast Recipes

1. Curried Tofu Scramble

Prep ten minutes/cook twenty minutes/press tofu thirty minutes/serves four

Ingredients:

SAUCE

.25 teaspoon salt

.25 teaspoon garam masala

.25 teaspoon turmeric

.25 teaspoon paprika

.25 teaspoon coriander

.5 teaspoon cumin

.25 teaspoon garlic powder

.5 teaspoon curry powder

SCRAMBLE

Spinach, rough chopped, three cups

Tofu, firm, block

Mushrooms, sliced, six ounces

Red bell pepper, diced and cleaned, one large

Onion, diced, one half medium

Vegetable broth, one tablespoon (or use olive oil or water)

Press and drain the block of tofu for thirty minutes before beginning the recipe.

Cook the onion in the vegetable broth for five minutes, then add the red peppers and the mushrooms and cook an additional ten minutes. Shove the cooked vegetables to one half of the skillet and put the tofu in the other half, breaking it into little chunks. Cook for five minutes. While the tofu is cooking dump all of the seasoning ingredients into a bowl and whip until smooth and well mixed. Dump this mix over the ingredients in the skillet and mix all together. Add in the greens, cook for five more minutes, and serve.

Nutrition: Calories 118, Carbs 8 grams, Protein 11 grams, Fat 4 grams

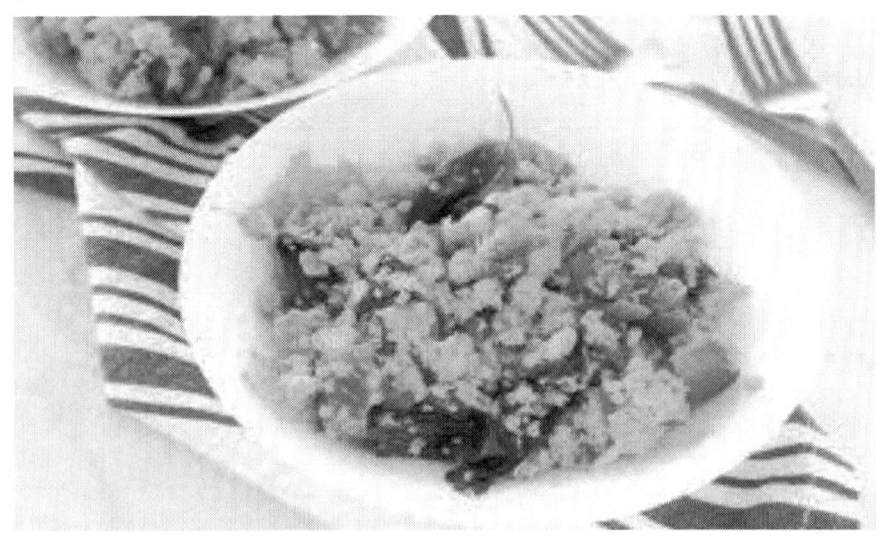

2. Maple Oatmeal

Prep five min/cook twenty min/serves four

Ingredients:
Maple flavoring, one teaspoon
Cinnamon, .5 teaspoon
Stevia powder, .25 teaspoon
Chia seeds, four tablespoons
Almond milk, three ounces
Coconut flakes, unsweetened, .25 cup
Sunflower seeds, three tablespoons
Pecans, .5 cup
Walnuts, .5 cup

Pulse the sunflower seeds, pecans, and walnuts in a food processor to crumble. If you do not have a food processor to use, then put them in a plastic bag, cover it with a towel, lay it on a cutting board, and beat it with a hammer.

Place the crushed nuts with the rest of the ingredients into a large pot and simmer over low heat for thirty minutes. Stir often so the chia seeds do not stick to the bottom. Serve garnished with fresh fruit or a sprinkle of cinnamon if desired.

Nutrition: Calories 374, 3.2 grams carbs, 9.25 grams protein, 34.59 grams fat

3. Scrambled Eggs with Cheese

Prep two min/cook three min/serve one

Ingredients:

Salt, .25 teaspoon

Black pepper, .5 teaspoon

Olive oil or butter, one tablespoon

Cheddar or Monterrey Jack cheese, .5 cup grated

Eggs, two

Warm the butter or the oil over medium heat. Crack the eggs into a small bowl and salt and pepper, mix well. Pout this mixture into the skillet and scramble until desired firmness, mixing often and well. When the eggs are almost done to your taste dump the cheese on top, cook two more minutes, and serve.

Nutrition: Calories 458, 2 grams carbs, 25.4 grams protein, 39 grams fat

4. Egg Breakfast Muffins

Prep five minutes/cook twenty minutes/serves six

Ingredients:

Curry powder, two teaspoons

Salt, .5 teaspoon

Cheddar cheese, two ounces

Spinach, .5 cup

Eggs, six

Cherry tomatoes, four

Spring onions, three

Red bell pepper, one cleaned

Heat the oven to 390. Dice the tomatoes, onions, and pepper and place them in a mixing bowl. Finely chop the cleaned spinach and then add it to the diced veggies. Add in the salt, curry powder, and eggs. Spoon the egg mixture evenly into six cups on a muffin tray. Bake for twenty minutes.

Nutrition: Calories 259, 11 grams carbs, 20 grams protein, 14 grams fat

5. Tomato Omelet

Prep two min/cook eight min/serves one

Ingredients:
Black pepper, .5 teaspoon
Salt, .25 teaspoon
Cheese, any type, .25 cup shred
Basil, fresh, .5 cup
Cherry tomatoes, .5 cup
Olive oil, two tablespoons
Eggs, two

Chop the tomatoes into small pieces. Fry the tomatoes in the oil for two to three minutes. Set the tomatoes to the side and wipe the pan clean.

In a small bowl mix the eggs well with the pepper and the salt. Dump the egg mixture into the pan and use a spatula to gently work around the edges under the omelet, letting it fry for three minutes.

When just the center third of the egg mix is still runny put on the cheese, basil, and tomatoes. Fold over half of the omelet onto the other half. Cook two more minutes and serve.

Nutrition: Calories 342, 8 grams carbs, 20 grams protein, 25.3 grams fat

6. Mediterranean Breakfast Burrito

Prep fifteen minutes/cook five minutes/serves six

Ingredients:

Salsa for garnish

Refried beans, canned, .75 cup

Feta cheese, .5 cup

Tomatoes, chopped, three tablespoons

Black olives, sliced, three tablespoons

Spinach, two cups, wash and dry

Eggs, six

Tortillas, ten inches, low carb, six

Scramble the eggs for five minutes in one tablespoon of butter. Stir in the tomatoes, black olives, and spinach and cook another five minutes, stirring constantly. Smear two tablespoons of the refried beans on each tortilla and top with the egg mix. Wrap each burrito and grill for five minutes on a griddle or in an electric skillet. Serve with salsa.

Nutrition: Calories 252, 19 grams carbs, 14 grams protein, 11 grams fat

7. Banana Pancakes

Prep three minutes/cook seven minutes/serves one

Ingredients:
Eggs, two
Banana, one

Cream together the eggs and the banana. Fry in melted butter over low heat.

Nutrition: Calories 231, 15 grams carbs, 12 grams protein, 9 grams fat

8. Chia Breakfast Pudding

Prep three min/serves two

Ingredients:
Almond butter, one tablespoon
Coconut milk, .75 cup
Cinnamon, .5 teaspoon

Vanilla, one teaspoon

Cold coffee, .75 cup

Chia seeds, four tablespoons

Mix all of the ingredients well and pour into a container, cover well and refrigerate overnight.

Nutrition: Calories 282, 5 grams carbs, 5.9 grams protein, 24 grams fat

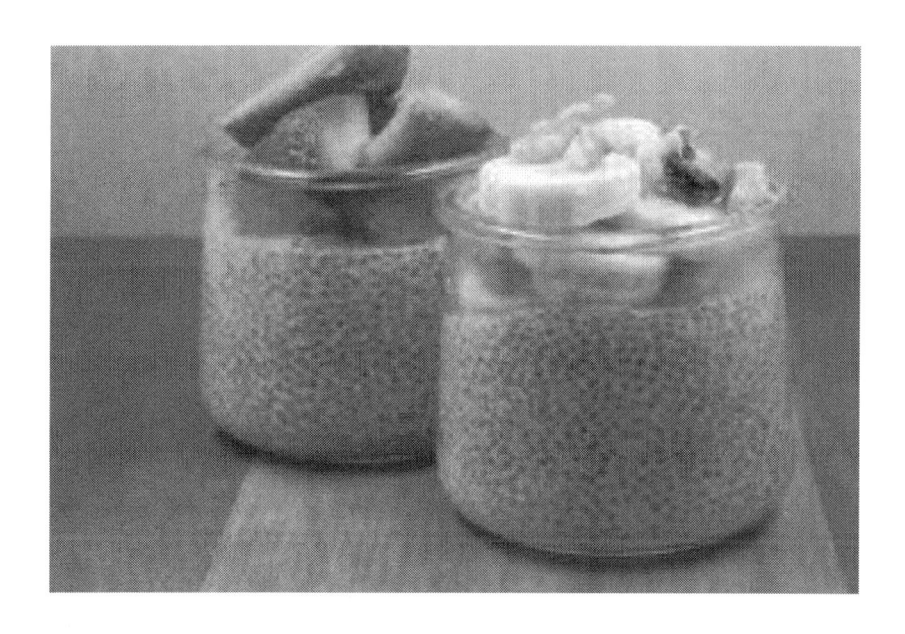

9. Five Ingredient Baked Pancake

Prep five min/cook fifteen min/serves eight

Bisquick, two cups

Almond milk, one and one half cup

Egg, one

Olive oil, .5 cup

For serving: fresh berries

Heat oven to 425. Use pan spray to coat a nine by thirteen baking pan. Make a batter of the oil, egg, milk, and Bisquick. Dump the batter into the baking pan and bake for fifteen minutes. Cut into squares and top with berries.

Nutrition: Calories 201, 23 grams carbs, 4.6 grams protein, 10 grams fat

10. Baked Eggs with Tomato and Spinach

Prep five minutes/cook twenty minutes/serves two

Ingredients:

Eggs, two

Salt, .5 teaspoon

Black pepper, .5 teaspoon

Red pepper flakes, one teaspoon

Basil, fresh, chop, .5 cup

Balsamic vinegar, two tablespoons

Olive oil, one tablespoon

Cheddar cheese, .5 cup

Onion, small, one

Tomatoes, four medium

Spinach, two cups

Heat oven to 400. Chop the tomatoes and dice the onions and mix together, and then add in the spinach. Mix in everything else except the eggs and stir together well. Spoon this mix into two pans that are oven safe and make a small indent in the middle. Crack the eggs, adding one to each pan. Bake for twenty minutes.

Nutrition: Calories 237, 10 grams carbs, 14 grams protein, 14 grams fat

11. Peppers and Onions Scrambled Eggs

Prep five min/cook five min/serve two

Ingredients:

Cilantro, fresh, .3 cup

Cheddar cheese, shredded, .5 cup

Eggs, four

Black pepper, .5 teaspoon

Salt, .5 teaspoon

Onion, diced, .5 cup

Red bell pepper, one diced

Olive oil, one tablespoon

Fry the onions and the peppers in the olive oil for five minutes. While they are frying beat the eggs well in a small bowl. Cook the beaten eggs in the skillet until they reach desired doneness, stirring often. When the eggs are almost done drop in the cheese and cilantro, mix well and serve.

Nutrition: Calories 369. 14 grams carbs, 20 grams protein, 25.8 grams fat

12. Avocado and Poached Egg

Prep two min/cook ten min/serves one

Ingredients:
Black pepper, .25 teaspoon
Salt, .25 teaspoon
Egg, one
Avocado, one half mashed

Mash the avocado half and spoon it onto a plate. Poach the egg and lay it on top of the mashed avocado.

Nutrition: Calories 407, 7 grams carbs, 15 grams protein, 23 grams fat

13. Spinach Mozzarella Frittata

Prep fifteen min/cook twenty min/serves four to six

Ingredients:
Salt, .5 teaspoon
Mozzarella cheese, shredded, one cup
Onion, .5 cup diced
Spinach, one cup diced
Almond milk, .5 cup
Eggs, eight
Olive oil, two tablespoons

Heat oven to 450. Fry the onions and the spinach in the olive oil for five minutes. While this is frying beat the eggs, milk, and salt in a bowl. Place the spinach onion mix into a greased nine by nine baking dish. Pour the eggs over the spinach mix and cover with the shredded cheese. Bake for twenty minutes.

Nutrition: Calories 315, 7 grams carbs, 22 grams protein, 22 grams fat

14. Baked Italian Skillet Eggs

Prep five min/cook ten min/serves two

Ingredients:
Parmesan cheese, grated, .25 cup
Mozzarella cheese, six ounces shredded
Eggs, four
Black pepper, .5 teaspoon
Salt, .5 teaspoon
Diced tomatoes, one twenty-eight ounce can
Red pepper flakes, .25 teaspoon
Garlic, minced, two tablespoons
Olive oil, one tablespoon

Fry the garlic and red pepper flakes in the olive oil for two minutes. Dump in the can of tomatoes with the juice and add the pepper and the salt. Simmer until the mix begins to bubble. Cook for five more minutes. Make four holes with the back of a spoon and crack one egg into each of the wells. Sprinkle both kinds of cheese over the mix and cook for ten minutes.

Nutrition: Calories 620, 15 grams carbs, 42 grams protein, 35 grams fat

15. Huevos Rancheros

Prep fifteen min/cook fifteen min/serves four

Ingredients:
Cilantro, fresh chopped, .25 cup
Feta cheese, crumbled, .25 cup
Eggs, four
Tomatoes, one large diced
Jalapeno pepper, one diced
Tomato paste, one tablespoon
Salt, .5 teaspoon
Cumin, ground, one teaspoon
Oregano, dried, one teaspoon
Garlic powder, one tablespoon
Onion, chopped, .25 cup
Olive oil, one tablespoon + one tablespoon

Cook the garlic and the onions in one tablespoon of olive oil for five minutes, stirring frequently. Add in the jalapeno, tomato paste, salt, oregano, and cumin and mix well for one minute. Pour in the diced tomatoes and simmer for four minutes. In another skillet heat the other tablespoon of olive oil and fry the eggs for five minutes turning once. Place spoons of the warm sauce on a plate and top with one fried egg, then sprinkle the eggs with the cilantro and the feta cheese.

Nutrition: Calories 198, 15 grams carbs, 12 grams protein, 8.9 grams fat

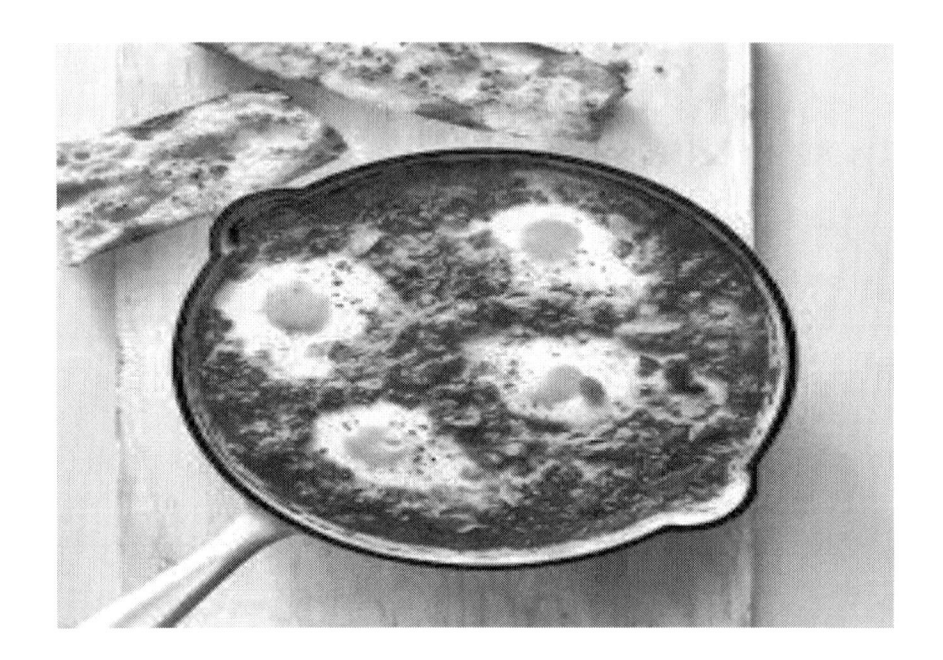

16. Baked Avocado Eggs

Prep ten min/cook fifteen min/serves four

Ingredients:

Parsley, fresh chop, .25 cup

Black pepper, .5 teaspoon

Salt, .25 teaspoon

Eggs, four

Olive oil, two tablespoons

Avocados, two

Heat oven to 375. Peel and slice the avocados and remove the pits. Slice a thin edge off the outside of each half so they will sit and not roll over. Brush on the olive oil to the inside of the avocado halves. Crack one egg into the center of each avocado half and season with salt and pepper. Bake fifteen minutes and sprinkle on the parsley to serve.

Nutrition: Calories 260, 8 grams carbs, 9 grams protein, 23 grams fat

17. Sweet Potato Hash Egg Muffin

Prep ten min/cook fifteen min/serves eight

Ingredients:

Salt and pepper

Eggs, eight

Garlic powder, .5 tablespoons

Cheddar cheese, .25 cup

Sweet potato, one small, grated

Heat oven to 375. Use lard to grease the cups of a muffin pan or use paper cups. Use a cheese grated to grate the sweet potato.

Mix in a bowl the garlic powder, cheddar cheese, and sweet potato. Scoop out one tablespoon of this mix for each of eight cups in the muffin pan. Then break one egg into each cup. Bake these for twelve to sixteen minutes or until the egg is cooked the way you prefer.

Nutrition: Calories 103, 4 grams carbs, 8 grams protein, 6 grams fat

18. Baked Scrambled Eggs

Prep ten min/cook twenty min/serves eight

Ingredients:
Chives, chopped, .5 cup
Salt, .5 teaspoon
Black pepper, .5 teaspoon
Almond milk, .5 cup
Eggs, eight
Butter, four tablespoons
Kale, one cup chop fine
Tomato, one cup diced

Heat oven to 350. Put the butter into a nine by thirteen baking pan and set the pan in the oven while it heats to easily melt the butter.

Tilt the pan different ways to cover the bottom with the butter. Use a large bowl to mix all of the ingredients well and pour them into the pan on top of the melted butter. Bake for sixteen to twenty minutes or until the eggs has cooked to your preferred doneness. Sprinkle the chopped chives on top and serve.

Nutrition: Calories 115, 5 grams carbs, 8.5 grams protein, 7.2 grams fat

19. Vegetable Quiche

Prep twenty-five min/cook one hour/serves six

Ingredients:
Parmesan cheese, grated, two tablespoons
Cheddar cheese, .75 cup
Salt, .5 teaspoon
Black pepper, one teaspoon
Almond milk, .5 cup
Eggs, four
Thyme, ground, one tablespoon
Garlic, two cloves minced
Orange bell pepper, one, cleaned and diced
Zucchini, peeled and sliced, one cup (one large)
Squash, peeled and sliced, one cup (one large)

Onion, diced fine, .5 cup

Olive oil, two tablespoons

Heat oven to 350. Fry the thyme, minced garlic, bell pepper, onion, squash, and zucchini for five minutes stirring often. While this is frying beat the black pepper, salt, and milk with the egg until well mixed. Pour the fried veggies into a greased nine by nine baking dish and top with the cheddar cheese. Cover this with the egg mix and then the parmesan cheese. Bake for fifty minutes and then let the quiche cool for ten minutes before you cut it.

Nutrition: Calories 240, 11 grams carbs, 12 grams protein, 9 grams fat

20. Egg Drop Soup

Prep five minutes/cook ten minutes/serves one

Ingredients:

Green onion, one sliced thin for garnish

Egg, one

Ginger, ground, .25 teaspoon

Garlic, powdered, .25 teaspoon

Black pepper, .25 teaspoon

Vegetable broth, one cup

Mix the seasonings into the broth until well mixed. Use a whisk in a bowl to beat the egg, saving the whisk. Bring broth to a simmer in a pan over medium heat. As soon as the broth is simmering use the whisk to stir the broth around until it makes a whirlpool effect and then slowly pour the egg in while you continue stirring. Once all the egg is stirred in remove the pan from the stove and pour the soup into a large mug and drop in the green onions.

Nutrition: Calories 65, 5.3 grams carbs, 2.8 grams protein, 2 grams fat

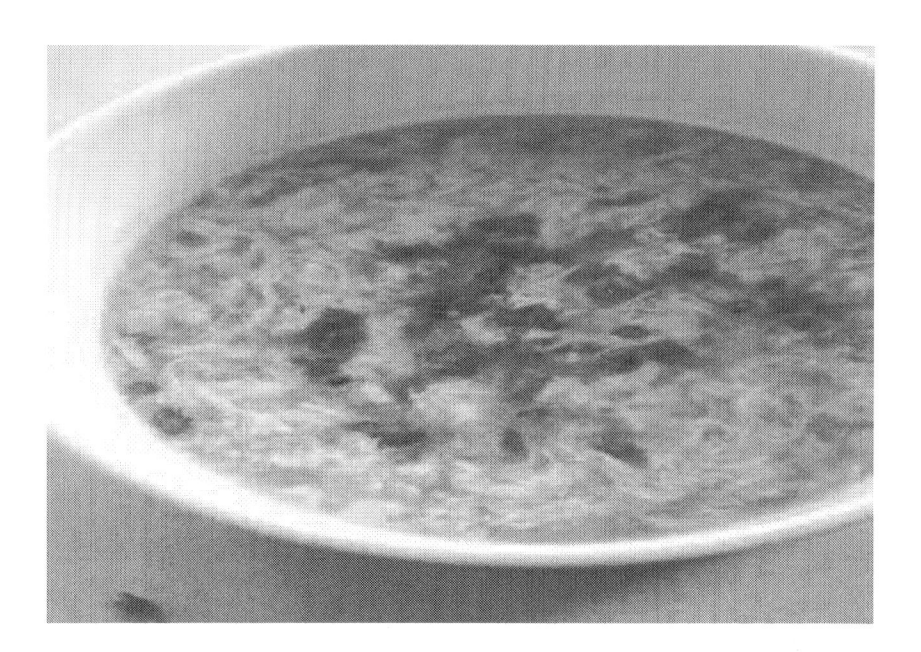

21. Mushroom Sandwich with Eggs and Greens

Prep forty-five minutes/cook forty-five min/serves four

Ingredients:
Tomato, one large sliced into four slices
Black pepper, .5 teaspoon
Salt, .5 teaspoon
Olive oil, one tablespoon
Portobello mushroom caps, four large with gills removed
Eggplant, four slices
Lemon juice, one teaspoon
Mayonnaise, .25 cup
Garlic, one clove minced
Arugula or spinach, two cups, cleaned and chopped and cooked as desired
Eggs, four

Mix the lemon juice, garlic, and mayonnaise in a small bowl and set to the side. Cover the mushroom caps and the rounds of eggplant with olive oil and grill in a large skillet for five minutes each side. Spread one teaspoon of the mayonnaise mixture on each mushroom cap and top with the rounds of eggplant and the slices of tomato. Fry the eggs until the desired doneness and lay them gently on top of the tomato. Drizzle on top any remaining mayonnaise mixture if desired and serve with a side of greens.

Nutrition: Calories 289, 15 grams carbs, 10 grams protein, 11 grams fat

22. Punjabi Egg Curry

Prep ten min/cook twenty min/serves two

Ingredients:

Water, .5 cup

Tomatoes, one cup diced

Chili powder, .25 teaspoon

Turmeric powder, .25 teaspoon

Garam masala, one teaspoon

Paprika, one teaspoon

Cumin, powdered, one teaspoon

Salt, one teaspoon

Coriander, powder, two teaspoons

Garlic, three cloves minced

Onion, one medium diced

Butter or ghee, two tablespoons

Eggs, six, hard-boiled, cooled, and peeled

For two minutes fry the onion and ginger in the ghee or the butter. Pour in the tomatoes, water, and the spices, and cook for five minutes. Simmer this mix for ten minutes and then add in the eggs, stirring often for five more minutes and serve.

Nutrition: Calories 156, 3 grams carbs, 7 grams protein, 13 grams fat

23. Eggs with Brussel Sprouts

Prep five min/cook twenty min/serves two

Ingredients:
Salt, .25 teaspoon
Black pepper, .5 teaspoon
Eggs, two
Brussel sprouts, grated, two cups
Butter or olive oil, two tablespoons

Fry the grated Brussel sprouts in the oil or butter for six to nine minutes until slightly soft and just beginning to brown. Make two holes in the cooked sprouts with the back of a spoon and break one egg into each well. Cook for five more minutes. Sprinkle on the pepper and the salt as desired and serve.

Nutrition: Calories 347, 15 grams carbs, 20 grams protein, 16 grams fat

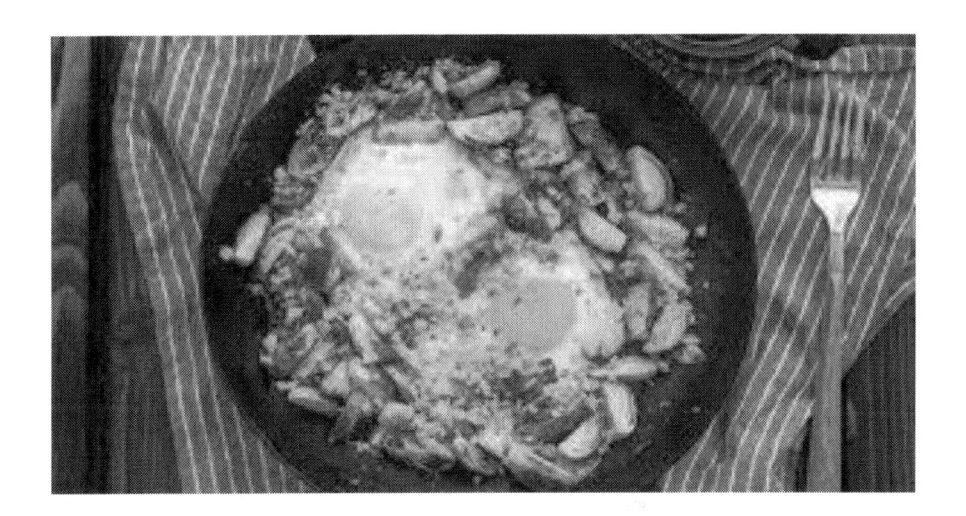

24. Cinnamon Custard

Prep twenty min/cook thirty min/serves six

Ingredients:

Vanilla extract, .5 teaspoon

Salt, .25 teaspoon

Sugar substitute, .5 cup

Egg yolks, two

Eggs, whole, two
Cinnamon, one teaspoon
Heavy cream, two cups

Heat oven to 300. Mix the cinnamon into the cream and simmer over low heat until the cream just begins to let off steam, then remove from the heat. Beat together the egg yolks, eggs, salt, and sugar substitute. While stirring this mixture constantly use a large spoon or ladle to pour in the heavy cream in small amounts, and then add the vanilla. Pour the mix into a round two-quart baking pan and bake for thirty-five to forty minutes (the custard will still be slightly loose just in the center). Serve this dish either warm or cold.

Nutrition: Calories 325, 4.9 grams carbs, 4.6 grams protein, 32.5 grams fat

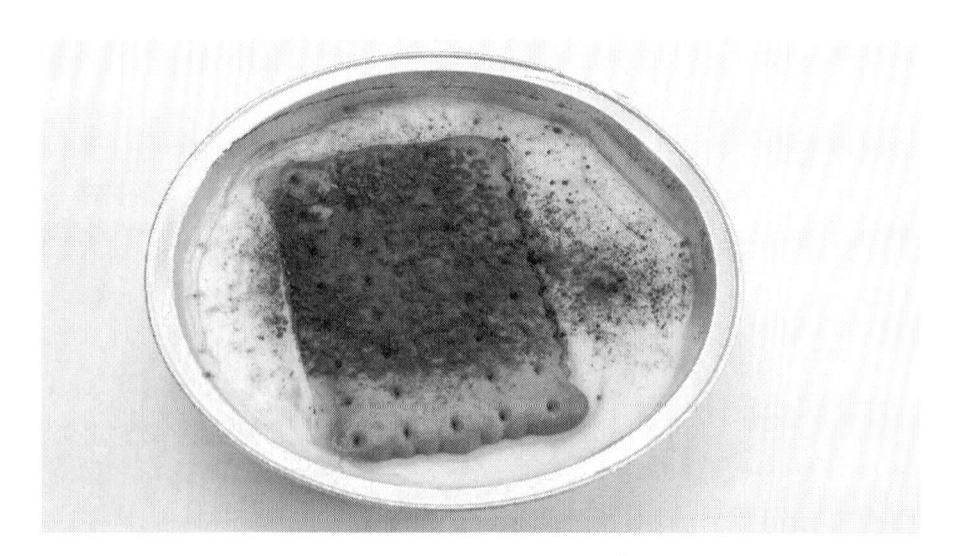

25. Cream Cheese Pancakes

Prep three min/cook nine minutes/serves one

Ingredients:

Cinnamon, .5 teaspoon

Eggs, two

Cream cheese, two ounces

Butter, two tablespoons for frying

Cream together all ingredients. This will be easier to do if the cream cheese has been allowed to soften slightly. Use the batter to make four pancakes cooked in the butter.

Nutrition: Calories 344, 3 grams carbs, 17 grams protein, 29 grams fat

Chapter 7: Lunch and Dinner Recipes

1. Cauliflower Rice and Mushroom Risotto

Prep twenty minutes/cook thirty minutes/serves six

Ingredients:

Black pepper, one teaspoon

Salt, .5 teaspoon

Parsley, fresh, chopped, two tablespoons

Parmesan cheese, grated, .5 cup

Heavy cream, one cup

Cauliflower, riced, four cups

Vegetable broth, two cups divided

Mushrooms, button, one cup sliced thin

Shallot, one large, minced

Onion, one small, well diced

Garlic, minced, six cloves

Olive oil, two tablespoons

Butter, two tablespoons

Add the olive oil and the butter together in one pan and fry the shallot, onion, and garlic for five minutes. Pour in one cup of the vegetables broth and the mushrooms and cook for five more minutes. To this mix and the other cup of vegetable broth and the riced cauliflower, cooking for ten minutes while stirring often. Pour in the heavy cream, salt, pepper, parsley, and the parmesan cheese and turn the heat under the pot to low. Simmer this for ten to fifteen minutes or until the mix is thickened.

Nutrition: Calories 297, 7.5 grams carbs, 7 grams protein, 26 grams fat

2. Grilled Eggplant Roll-Ups

Prep five min/cook eight min/serves eight

Ingredients:
Olive oil, two tablespoons
Basil, fresh, chopped, two tablespoons
Tomato, one large
Mozzarella cheese, four ounces
Eggplant, one medium

After cutting off both of the ends of the eggplant slice it into strips the long way about a quarter inch thick. Slice the tomato and the mozzarella very thinly and set to the side. Brush the olive oil onto the slices of eggplant and grill them in a skillet for three minutes on each side. When both sides are grilled lay a slice of cheese and a slice of tomato on each zucchini slice. Sprinkle all with the black pepper and the basil, then let grill for two to three minutes until the cheese begins to soften. Remove the slices from the skillet and lie on a plate, then carefully roll each slice as far as it will roll.

Nutrition: Calorie 59, 4 grams carbs, 3 grams protein, 3 grams fat

3. Eggplant Gratin with Feta Cheese

Prep fifteen min/cook forty min/serves six

Ingredients:
Salt, .5 teaspoon
Black pepper, .5 teaspoon
Olive oil, three tablespoons
Tomato sauce, .5 cup
Gruyere cheese, .75 cup,
Basil, fresh chop, .25 cup
Chives, chopped, one tablespoon
Thyme, chopped, one teaspoon
Feta cheese, crumbled, three ounces
Heavy cream, one cup
Eggplant, two, half-inch slices

Heat oven to 375. Lay the eggplant slices on a baking pan and coat with olive oil and sprinkle on pepper and salt and bake the slices for twenty minutes. While they are baking put the Feta cheese and heavy cream in a pot and let boil. Remove the cooking pot from the heat and stir in the chives and thyme and set to the side. Spread all of the tomato sauce on the bottom of a nine by thirteen baking pan and lay the eggplant slices over the bottom.

Cover the slices with the Gruyere cheese and the basil. Add another layer with the rest of the eggplant and cover all with the heavy cream mixture.

Bake for twenty minutes.

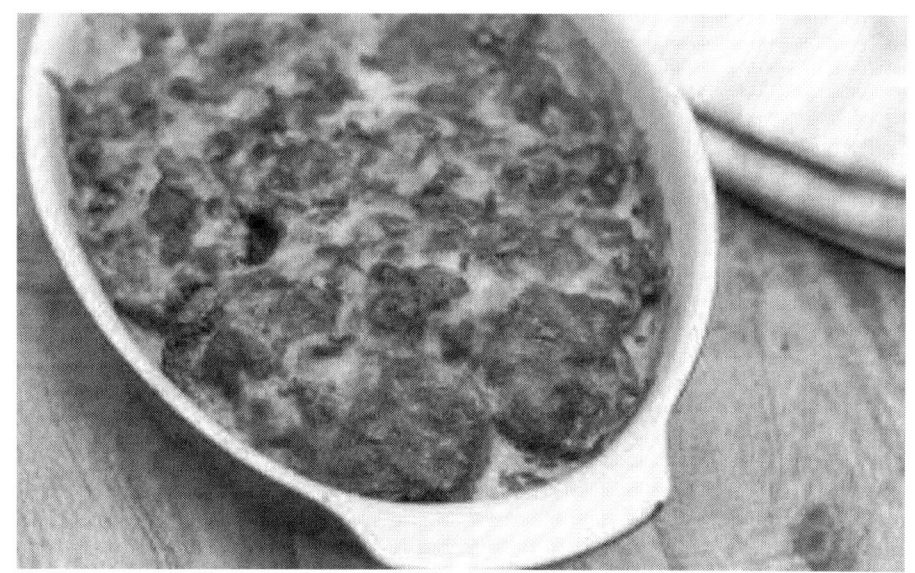

Nutrition: Calories 302, 14 grams carbs, 9.4 grams protein, 24.3 grams fat

4. Stuffed Zucchini with Marinara and Goat Cheese

Prep ten min/cook ten min/serves four

Ingredients:
Parsley, chopped, to garnish with
Marinara sauce, one cup
Goat cheese, sixteen ounces
Zucchini, medium-sized, four

Heat oven to 400. Cut the zucchinis in half the long way and cut out the seeds. Sprinkle on pepper and salt to taste. Place four ounces of goat cheese in each zucchini and cover with one-fourth cup of marinara sauce. Bake for ten minutes.

Nutrition: Calories 81, 6 grams carbs, 3 grams protein, 5 grams fat

5. Herb and Halloumi Tomato Salad

Prep ten min/serves four

Ingredients:
Tomatoes, sliced, one pound

Salt, .25 teaspoon

Black pepper, .5 teaspoon

Halloumi cheese, one-half pound sliced

Parsley, fresh, chopped, two tablespoons

Lemon juice, one tablespoon

Olive oil, two tablespoons

Basil, fresh chop, two tablespoons

Use the lemon juice, pepper, and salt to season the slices of tomato. Place the slices on four serving plates and top with slices of halloumi cheese and drizzle the cheese with the olive oil. Use the basil and the parsley to garnish with and serve.

Nutrition: Calories 196, 8 grams carbs, 9 grams protein, 15 grams fat

6. Greek Fattoush Salad

Prep fifteen min/serves six

DRESSING

Olive oil, .3 cup

Red wine vinegar, two tablespoons

Black pepper, .50 teaspoon

Salt, .25 teaspoon

Oregano, .25 teaspoon

Garlic, one clove minced

SALAD

Salt, .25 teaspoon

Feta cheese, .75 cup crumble

Black olives, .5 cup slice

Parsley, fresh, .5 cup chop

Red onion, one small thin slice

Cucumber, one peeled, quarter and slice

Cherry tomatoes, one cup slice

Yellow bell pepper, diced

Romaine lettuce, four cups chop

Olive oil, two tablespoons

Mix all of the ingredients that are listed for the dressing in a bowl and set to the side. Use a larger bowl to mix the lettuce with the cucumber, tomatoes, bell pepper, onion, olives, and parsley tossing gently until well mixed. Dribble on top the chunks of feta cheese and serve with the dressing on the side.

Nutrition: Calories 294, 11 grams carbs, 15 grams protein, 12 grams fat

7. Veggie Stuffed Peppers

Prep thirty min/serves six

Ingredients:

Greek yogurt, .5 cup

Rice wine vinegar, two tablespoons

Parsley, fresh, .25 cup chopped

Celery washed and diced four stalks

Cherry tomatoes, cut in quarters, one cup

Green bell peppers, three, cleaned and cut in half across the middle

Dijon mustard, three tablespoons

Salt, .25 teaspoon

Black pepper, .5 teaspoon

Scallions, one bunch, cleaned and sliced

Cucumber, one half, peeled and diced

In one bowl mix together the yogurt, rice wine vinegar, mustard, salt, and pepper. Add in the celery, tomatoes, scallions, and cucumbers and mix gently but well. Use a spoon to stuff this mix into the pepper halves.

Nutrition: Calories 117, 9 grams carbs, 7 grams protein, 3 grams fat

8. Eggplant Chickpea Stew

Prep thirty min/cook fifteen min/serves two

Ingredients:
Olive oil, three tablespoons
Black pepper, .5 teaspoon
Salt, .25 teaspoon
Garlic powder, two tablespoons
Chickpeas, fourteen ounces can drain and rinse
Cilantro, one tablespoon
Eggplant, one peel, and cube
Onion, one diced fine
Tomatoes, one fourteen ounces can be drained
Hot sauce, any brand, one tablespoon

Fry the eggplant, onion, garlic, salt, and pepper in the olive oil for five minutes. Pour in the tomatoes, chickpeas, and hot sauce; mix well and simmer for fifteen minutes.

Nutrition: Calories 350, 16 grams carbs, 12 grams protein, 10 grams fat

9. Springtime Greek Soup

Prep fifteen min/cook thirty min/serves six

Ingredients:
Vegetable broth, six cups
Olive oil, two tablespoons
Onion, diced, one small
Lemon juice, three tablespoons
Asparagus, chopped, one cup
Carrots, diced small, one cup
Dill, fresh, chopped, .25 cup
Black pepper, .5 teaspoon
Salt, .5 teaspoon
Chives, fresh, chopped, .5 cup

Fry the dill and onion for five minutes in the olive oil. Pour in the vegetable broth, carrots, and asparagus and simmer for twenty minutes. After twenty minutes stir in the lemon juice and the chives and serve.

Nutrition: Calories 250,12 grams carbs, 18 grams protein, 9.7 grams fa

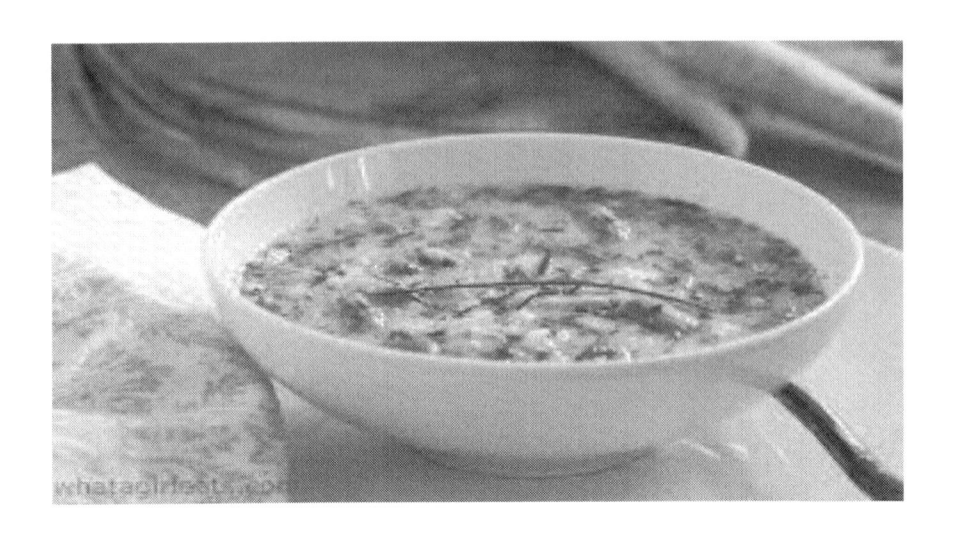

10. Spicy Lentil Soup*

Prep twenty min/cook fifty min/serves eight

Ingredients:

Olive oil, three tablespoons

Yellow onion, one chopped fine

Parsley, fresh, chopped, .5 cup

Celery, Fine chop, .5 cup

Ginger, two tablespoons minced

Cilantro, chopped, .5 cup

Cinnamon, one tablespoon

Paprika, one tablespoon

Lentils, dry, one cup

Tomato, two large, cleaned and diced

Chickpeas, one can fifteen-ounce drain and rinse

Black pepper, one teaspoon

Salt, .5 teaspoon

Vegetable broth, seven cups

Fry the celery, garlic, onion, ginger, and carrots in the olive oil for eight to ten minutes, stirring often. Add in the cinnamon, turmeric, salt, pepper, and paprika and cook for five more minutes. Add the tomatoes and the vegetable broth and mix in well. Let the soup simmer for five minutes and then mix in the lentils, cilantro, chickpeas, and the parsley, then let the entire mix simmer for thirty minutes.

Lentils, in small quantities like this soup, are relatively low in carbs with only 3 grams per tablespoon.

Nutrition per two cups of soup: Calories 240, 20 grams carbs, 14 grams protein, 7.4 grams fat

11. Tomato and Red Pepper Soup

Prep fifteen min/cook forty-five min/serves four

Ingredients:

Black pepper, .5 teaspoon

Vegetable Broth, vegetable, two cups

Garlic, two cloves, peel and halve

Cayenne pepper, .25 teaspoon

Italian seasoning, .5 teaspoon

Olive oil, three tablespoons

Onion, one medium, cut in quarters

Paprika, ground, .5 teaspoon

Parsley, fresh, chop, .25 cup

Red bell peppers, two, seeded and diced

Salt, .25 teaspoon

Tomato paste, two tablespoons

Tomato, three, clean and dice

Heat oven to 425. Use a large mixing bowl to mix the tomatoes, red pepper, garlic, and onion, with the pepper, salt, and olive oil. Spread the veggies on a baking pan and bake not covered for forty-five minutes. Pour the vegetable broth into a pot and heat to boiling then turn the heat down and add in the roasted veggies, stir well and simmer for five minutes and serve.

Nutrition per one cup: Calories 150, 14 grams carbs, 4 grams protein, 4 grams fat

12. Zucchini Soup

Prep twenty min/cook forty min/serves eight

Ingredients:
Zucchini, three pounds
Olive oil, three tablespoons
Garlic, three cloves fine chop
Onion, one small diced fine
Vegetable broth, five cups
Black pepper, .5 teaspoon
Salt, .5 teaspoon
Basil, dried, .25 cup

Fry the garlic, onion, and zucchini for five minutes in hot olive oil. Add in the vegetable broth and let the mix simmer for fifteen minutes. Stir in the salt and the pepper. Remove three of the cups of the soup from the pot, making sure to get veggies with the broth, and mix it in a blender until it is smooth. Add this blended soup back into the pot and stir well until well mixed and serve.

Nutrition for one cup: Calories 79, 8.5 grams carbs, 2 grams protein, 5 grams fat

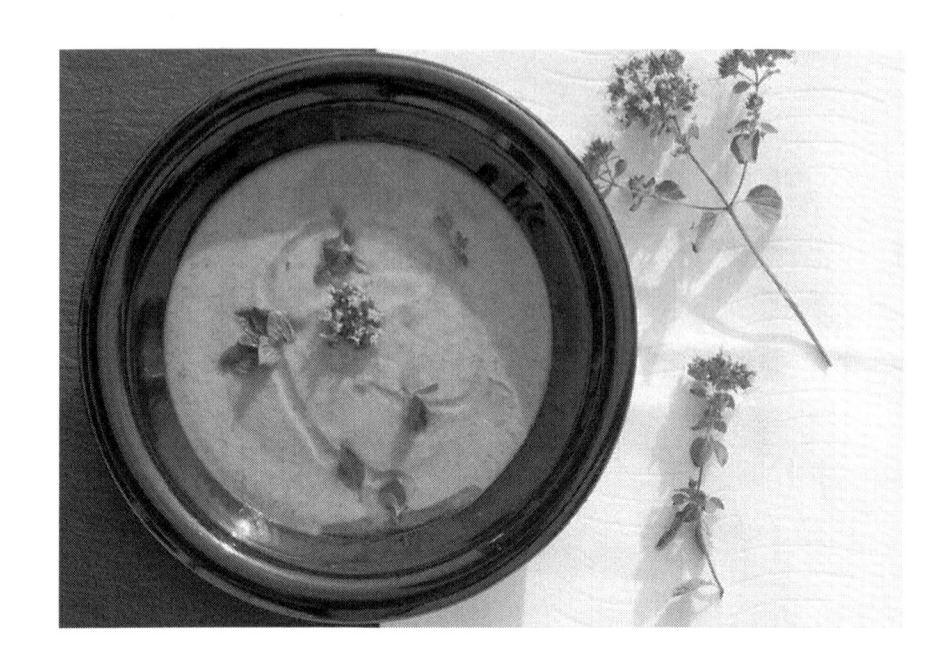

13. Tuscany Vegetable Soup

Prep fifteen min/cook thirty min/serves eight

Ingredients:

Parsley, fresh chopped for garnisSalt, .5 teaspoon

Black pepper, one teaspoon

Basil, one tablespoon chop fine

Kale, two cups chop

Tomato paste, two tablespoons

Vegetable broth, six cups

Tomatoes, two large diced small

Zucchini, one medium peeled and chopped
Celery, .5 cup chop
Carrot, .5 cup chop
Yellow onion, one medium diced
Garlic, four cloves minced
Olive oil, three tablespoons

Fry the onion and the garlic in the heated olive oil in a soup pot. Then add in the celery, carrots, and the zucchini and cook for ten minutes stirring frequently. Mix in well the tomatoes, pepper, and salt and cook two more minutes. Pour in the vegetable broth and the tomato paste and bring the whole mix to a boil. Turn the heat lower and let the mix simmer for fifteen minutes. Put in the parsley and the basil, remove the pot from the heat and let the soup sit for ten minutes. Garnish with fresh parsley and serve.
Nutrition per one cup: Calories 225, 12 grams carbs, 17 grams protein, 6 grams fat

14. Cheddar Cheese and Roast Cauliflower Soup

Prep time ten min/cook forty-five minutes/serves eight

Ingredients:
Olive oil, three tablespoons

Black pepper, one teaspoon

Salt, .5 teaspoon

Garlic powder, one tablespoon

Onion, one medium fine chop

Cauliflower, one full head chopped

Cheddar cheese, three cups

Vegetable broth, six cups

Heat oven to 400. Chop the cauliflower and coat with one tablespoon of the olive oil and toss with the salt, pepper, and olive oil. Bake the cauliflower on a cookie sheet for thirty minutes. Add the onions to the rest of the olive oil and fry them in a large pot for five minutes. Pour in the vegetable broth and the roasted cauliflower and cook for thirty minutes. Stir in the cheddar cheese until just melted and serve.

Nutrition per two cups: Calories 243, 8.3 grams carbs, 14 grams protein, 17 grams fat

15. Cabbage Soup

Prep twenty min/cook one hour/serves eight

Ingredients:

Thyme, crushed, one teaspoon

Black pepper, one teaspoon

Salt, .5 teaspoon

Crushed tomatoes, one twenty-eight ounce can

Tomato sauce, one eight ounce can

Celery, three stalks sliced

Carrots, three sliced thin

Green cabbage, one head, cored and chopped

Red cabbage, one-half head chopped

Vegetable broth, three cups

Onion, one chopped

Olive oil, two tablespoon

Fry onion in olive oil in a large skillet for five minutes. Stir in vegetable broth into the pot. Mix in crushed tomatoes, tomato sauce, beans, celery, carrots, and both cabbages and mix well. Stir in thyme and salt. Boil one minute, then lower heat and then simmer one hour.

Nutrition info: Calories 404, 14 grams carbs, 15 grams protein, 13 grams fat

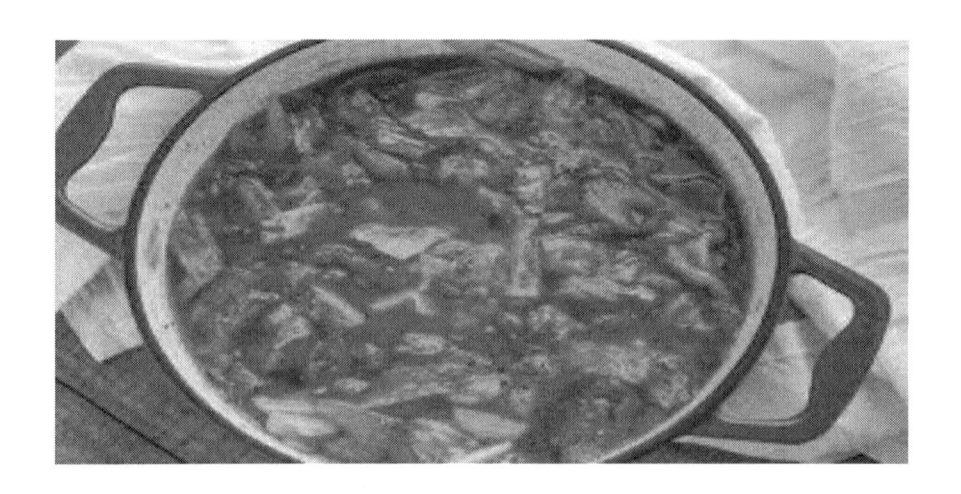

16. Nicoise Salad

Prep forty minutes/serves four

Ingredients:

DRESSING

Olive oil, three tablespoons

Lemon juice, two tablespoons

Water, one tablespoon

Garlic, one clove minced

Salt, .25 teaspoon

Black pepper, .5 teaspoon

SALAD

Eggs, hard-boiled, two sliced

Green beans, French style, four ounces

Olive oil, one tablespoon

Bibb lettuce, one large head

Red onion, thin sliced, .5 cup

Grape tomatoes, one cup

Basil leaves, chopped fine, .5 cup

Black olives, pitted, .5 cup

Salt, .5 teaspoon

Black pepper, one teaspoon

Blend in a small bowl all of the ingredients that are listed for the dressing until smooth and then place in the refrigerator while you assemble the salad. Place the green beans in boiling water and boil for three minutes, and then remove and drain. Put the Bibb lettuce evenly on four plates and top with equal amounts of the eggs, tomatoes, black olives, onions, and green beans. Serve the salad with sides of the cooled dressing.

Nutrition: Calories 350, 14 grams carbs, 22 grams protein, 10 grams fat

17. Sprout Wraps

Prep fifteen min/serves two

Ingredients:

Tortillas, low carb two large

Black pepper, one teaspoon

Salt, one teaspoon

Lemon juice, one tablespoon

Olive oil, one tablespoon

Parsley, .5 cup

Onion, green, two stalks

Cucumber, one sliced thin

Bean sprouts, one cup

Nutrition: Calories 226, 12 grams carbs, 10 grams protein, 3 grams fat

18. Cheesy Gratin Zucchini

Prep ten min/cook forty-five min/serves nine

Ingredients:

Heavy cream, .5 cup

Garlic powder, one tablespoon

Butter, two tablespoons

Pepper jack cheese, two cups shredded

Salt, .25 teaspoon

Black pepper, .25 teaspoon

White onion, one small, peel and slice thin

Zucchini, sliced, raw, four cups

Heat oven to 375. Use lard to grease a nine by nine baking dish. Lay one-third of the onion and the zucchini slice in the pan so they barely overlap, then sprinkle on pepper and salt and one half of the pepper jack cheese. Add another layer of the onion and zucchini slices seasoned with the pepper and the salt and sprinkled with the rest of the pepper jack cheese. Then lay on the remainder of the onions and the zucchini slices. Microwave for one minute the heavy cream, butter, and garlic powder just until the butter melts and mix it well, then pour it over the top layer of slices. Bake not covered for forty-five minutes.

Nutrition: Calories 230, 3 grams carbs, 8 grams protein, 20 grams fat

19. Cilantro Lime Coleslaw

Prep ten min/serves five

Ingredients:
Salt, .5 teaspoon
Water, .25 cup
Garlic, one clove, diced
Lime juice, two tablespoons
Cilantro, fresh leaves, .25 cup

Avocados, two

Coleslaw, ready-made in the bag, fourteen ounces

Chop the cilantro and the garlic until minced. Put them in a blender or a food processor with the water, avocados, and the lime juice and mix until creamy smooth. Mix the coleslaw mix in with this dressing and toss gently to mix it well. Store in the refrigerator at least one hour before eating.

Nutrition: Calories 119, 3.2 grams carbs, 2.2 grams protein, 8.9 grams fat

20. Caprese Tomatoes with Basil Dressing

Prep five min/cook thirty min/serves two to four

Ingredients:
DRESSING
Salt, .25 teaspoon
Olive oil, two tablespoons
Lemon juice, two tablespoons
Garlic powder, one tablespoon
Basil, dried, one teaspoon

TOMATOES
Basil, dried, one tablespoon

Mozzarella cheese, four thin slices

Salt, .25 teaspoon

Black pepper, .5 teaspoon

Balsamic vinegar, two tablespoons

Olive oil, one tablespoon

Tomatoes, ripe, four large

Heat oven to 350. Cut the core end out of the tomato and cut each tomato in half across. Lay the tomato halves on a cookie sheet with the inside up.

Coat each half with a mixture of the Balsamic Vinegar, olive oil, pepper, and salt. Bake the tomato halves for twenty-five minutes. Place one of the thin slices of mozzarella cheese on each tomato bottom half and bake for five more minutes. Place some crushed basil on each tomato and put the top half back on the bottom half. Dribble the dressing over the tomatoes to serve.

Nutrition: Calories 240, 1.9 grams carbs, 6.5 grams protein, 7.5 grams fat

21. Greek Collard wraps

Prep twenty min/serves four
Ingredients:

SAUCE

Black pepper, one teaspoon

Salt, .5 teaspoon

Dill, fresh, minced, two tablespoons

Cucumber, seeded and grated, .25 cup

Olive oil, two tablespoons

White vinegar, one tablespoon

Garlic powder, one teaspoon

Greek yogurt, full fat, plain, one cup

WRAP

Cherry tomatoes, four cuts in half

Feta cheese, block style, four ounces, cut in four one inch thick strips

Black olives, sliced, .25 cup

Purple onion, .5 cup diced fine

Red bell pepper, one half of one cut in julienne strips

Cucumber, one medium sized cut in julienne strips

Green collard leaves, four large

Place all of the ingredients listed for the sauce in a mixing bowl and mix well. Store the dressing in the refrigerator. Wash off the collard leaves and then cut off the stem from each leaf. Cover each leaf with two tablespoons of the sauce you just made. Layer all of the other ingredients in the middle of the collard leaf. Fold the leaf up like a burrito by first folding the ends in and then rolling the leaf until it is all rolled. Cut into slices and serve with more dressing for dipping.

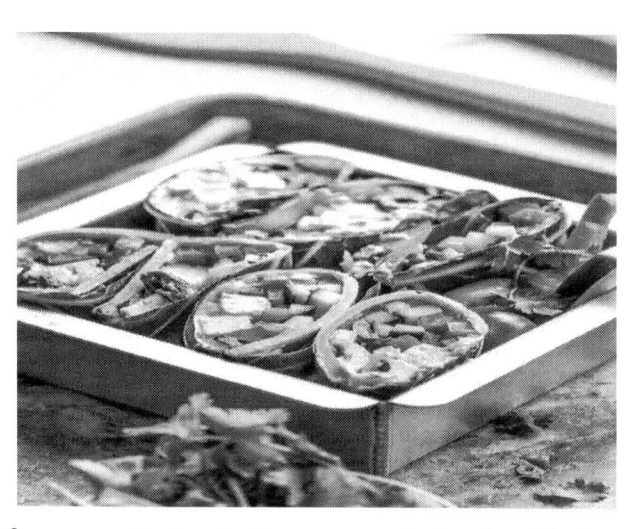

Nutrition per wrap: Calories 165, 7.36 grams carbs, 6.98 grams protein, 11.25 grams fat

22. Zucchini and Spinach Lasagna

Prep twenty min/cook fifty min/serves nine

Ingredients:
Parsley, chopped, one teaspoon
Mozzarella cheese, shredded, sixteen ounces

Zucchini, four medium, peeled and sliced long ways into thin slices

Parmesan cheese, grated, .5 cup

Egg, one large

Ricotta cheese, fifteen ounces

Spinach, three cups

Basil, chopped, one tablespoon

Salt, .5 teaspoon

Black pepper, one teaspoon

Crushed tomatoes, one twenty-eight ounce can

Tomato paste, two tablespoons

Garlic, four cloves, crushed

Onion, fine chop, .5 cup

Olive oil, one tablespoon

Heat oven to 375. Cook the onions and the garlic in the olive oil for five minutes. Stir in the salt, pepper, canned tomatoes, and the tomato paste. Simmer this sauce for twenty-five minutes. Stir in the spinach and the fresh basil as soon as you remove the pot from the heat. In a mixing bowl mix the egg, parmesan cheese, and the ricotta cheese. Lay the slices of zucchini on a cookie sheet and bake for ten minutes. Grease a nine by thirteen baking dish and spread a thin layer of the tomato sauce on the bottom of the dish. Cover the sauce with five or six slices of zucchini. Spoon some of the ricotta cheese mixes on top of the sliced zucchini and then sprinkle with mozzarella cheese. Use all of the ingredients as you keep on making layers. Cover the baking dish with aluminum foil and bake the lasagna for thirty minutes, then take off the foil and bake it for an additional fifteen minutes. Let the lasagna stand untouched for ten minutes before you cut it. Use the parsley to garnish.

23. Fried Goat Cheese with Charred Veggies

Prep ten min/cook fifteen min/serves two

Ingredients:
Olive oil, one tablespoon
Arugula, four cups, two cups per bowl
Portobello mushrooms, baby, .5 cup sliced
Red bell pepper, one medium size, cleaned and sliced into eight slices
Goat cheese, four ounces, cut into one-ounce pieces
Garlic, minced, one teaspoon
Onion flakes, one teaspoon
Sesame seeds, two tablespoons
Poppy seeds, two tablespoons

Mix together the garlic, onion flakes, sesame seeds, and poppy seeds in a bowl. Place each piece of goat cheese into this mix to cover both sides with the seed mixture. Heat a skillet over high heat and place the mushrooms and the peppers slices in it and char them on both sides. Place the mushrooms and the peppers in the bowls with the arugula. Add the goat cheese to the skillet and cook on each side for no more than one minute. Flip gently as this cheese melts quickly. Put the warm cheese slices in the salad bowls and dribble with the olive oil.

Nutrition per bowl: Calories 350, 7.08 grams carbs, 16 grams protein, 27 grams fat

24. Vegetarian Club Salad

Prep fifteen min/serves three

Ingredients:
Dijon mustard, one tablespoon
Cucumber, diced, one cup
Cherry tomatoes, .5 cup cut in half
Romaine lettuce, three cups cut into pieces
Swiss cheese, cubed, one cup
Eggs, hard-boiled, three sliced
Parsley, dried, one teaspoon
Onion powder, .5 teaspoon
Garlic powder, .5 teaspoon
Mayonnaise, two tablespoons
Sour cream, two tablespoons

Mix the mayonnaise, sour cream, and the herbs until well mixed to make the dressing for the salad. Create the salads in three bowls by mixing in layers the sliced egg, cheese cubes, and the fresh vegetables. Drop one spoon of Dijon mustard in the center of each salad. Serve with the already prepared dressing on the side.

Nutrition: Calories 330, 5 grams carbs, 17 grams protein, 27 grams fat

25. Spiral Zucchini and Grape Tomatoes

Prep five min/cook ten min/serve two

Ingredients:

Zucchini, one large cut in spirals

Basil, fresh, chopped, one tablespoon

Black pepper, one teaspoon

Salt, .5 teaspoon

Crushed red pepper flakes, .18 teaspoon

Grape tomatoes, one cup cut in half

Garlic, cloves, three minced

Olive oil, one tablespoon

Cook the minced garlic in the olive oil for one minute. Pour in the salt, pepper, red pepper flakes, and the tomatoes and mix well the lower the heat. Simmer this mix for fifteen minutes. Add the basil and the zucchini spiral noodles and turn the heat back up and cook for two minutes, stirring constantly.

Nutrition: Calories 117, 13 grams carbs, 4 grams protein, 5 grams fat

26. Cauliflower Fried Rice

Prep five min//cook ten min/serves four

Ingredients:
Toasted sesame oil, one teaspoon
Soy sauce, two tablespoons
Egg, one large beaten
Garlic, two cloves crushed
Green onion, .25 cup
Carrot, .25 cup chopped fine
Riced cauliflower, twelve ounces frozen or fresh
Olive oil, ghee, or butter, two tablespoons

Cook the riced cauliflower and the carrots in the oil or butter you choose to use for about five minutes, stirring sometimes. Stir in this mix the chopped green onion and the garlic and cook for one minute. Add the beaten egg to the rice mix and stir until the egg is scrambled throughout the rice, about two to three minutes. Just before serving mix in the soy sauce and the sesame oil.

Nutrition: Calories 114, 6 grams carbs, 4 grams protein, 8 grams fat

27. Cheesy Broccoli and Cauliflower Rice

Prep 5 min/cook 8 min/serves four

Ingredients:
Mascarpone cheese, .25 cup
Sharp cheddar cheese, shredded, .5 cup
Nutmeg, ground, .25 teaspoon
Garlic powder, .25 teaspoon
Black pepper, .5 teaspoon
Salt, .5 teaspoon
Butter, one tablespoon
Riced broccoli, one cup
Riced cauliflower, three cups

Use a microwave-safe bowl to mix the nutmeg, garlic powder, pepper, salt, butter, broccoli, and cauliflower and microwave on high temperature for four minutes then stir well. Microwave on high temperature for two more minutes. Mix in the cheddar cheese and microwave for an additional two minutes. Carefully remove the bowl from the microwave and mix in the mascarpone cheese and stir to mix well. Serve while very hot.

Nutrition for one cup: Calories 138, 5 grams carbs, 6 grams protein, 11 grams fat

28. Mediterranean Pasta

Prep ten min/cook fifteen min/serves four

Ingredients:
Feta cheese, .25 cup, crumbled
Parmesan cheese, .25 cup, shredded
Kalamata olives, ten cuts in half
Parsley, flat leaf, chopped, two tablespoons
Capers, two tablespoons
Tomatoes, diced, .5 cup
Salt, .5 teaspoon
Black pepper, one teaspoon
Garlic, five cloves, minced
Butter, two tablespoons
Olive oil, two tablespoons
Spinach, one cup, pack
Zucchini, two large cuts in a spiral slice

Fry together in the olive oil and the butter the pepper, salt, spinach, and the zucchini for ten minutes until the spinach wilts and the zucchini feels tender when stuck with a fork. Drain off any excess liquid. Add in the olives, parsley, capers, and tomatoes and mix well, cooking for another five minutes. Blend in the feta cheese and the parmesan cheese and serve immediately.

Nutrition: Calories 231, 6.5 grams carbs, 6.5 grams protein, 20 grams fat

29. Roast Baby Eggplant

Prep twenty min/cook forty-five min/serves four

Ingredients:

FOR SERVING

Salt, one teaspoon

Black pepper, one teaspoon

Olive oil, two tablespoons

Ricotta cheese, .5 cup

TO COOK

Black pepper, one teaspoon

Salt, one teaspoon

Olive oil, two tablespoons

Baby eggplant, eight

Heat oven to 350. Wipe off the eggplant and cut each one in half the long way. Lay them on a baking pan inside up and coat the insides with olive oil and sprinkle on pepper and salt. Bake the baby eggplant for forty-five minutes or until they become soft and brown slightly. Just before you serve them top each eggplant half with a teaspoon of the ricotta cheese and top that with the olive oil, pepper, and salt.

Nutrition per half an eggplant: Calories 44, 1 gram carbs, 1 gram protein, 4 grams fat

30. Squash and Sweet Potato Patties

Prep fifteen minutes/cook ten minutes/serves two

Ingredients:
Ghee, two tablespoons
Salt, .5 teaspoon
Black pepper, one teaspoon
Parsley, dried, .25 teaspoon
Cumin, ground, .25 teaspoon

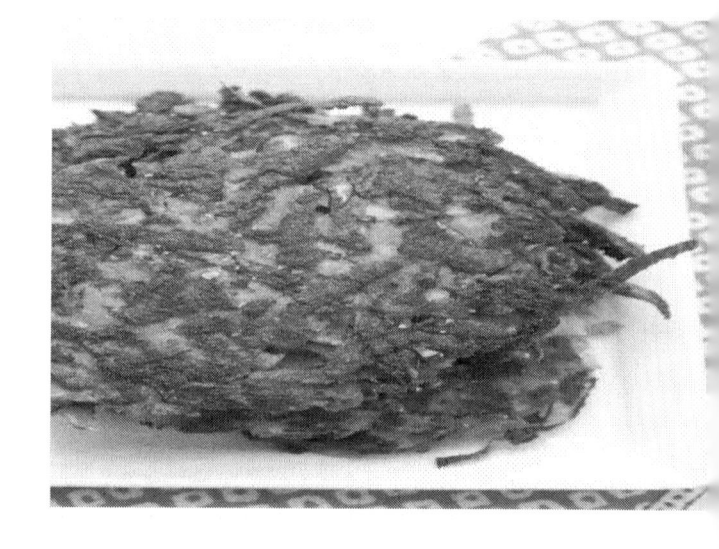

Garlic powder, .5 teaspoon

Egg, one, beaten

Sweet potato, shredded, one cup

Squash, shredded, one cup

Mix the beaten egg, sweet potato, and squash in a mixing bowl. Add in the spices and mix the ingredients well. Melt the ghee in a skillet and separate the mix into four equal portions. Drop the portions into the ghee and flatten slightly with a fork. Fry the patties for five minutes on each side and serve.

Nutrition per patty: Calories 112, 6 grams carbs, 3 grams protein, 9 grams fat

31. Chickpea Salad

Prep twenty min/serves four

Ingredients:

Salt, .5 teaspoon

Black pepper, one teaspoon

Lemon juice, two tablespoons

Olive oil, two tablespoons

Red onion, sliced thin, .5 cup

Parsley, fresh, chopped, .25 cup

Cucumber, chopped, one cup

Chickpeas, one cup drained and rinsed

Cherry tomatoes, red, one cup cut in halves

Cherry tomatoes, yellow, one cup cut in halves

Mix the tomatoes, cucumber, chickpeas, and onion together in a medium sized mixing bowl. Add in all of the seasonings to the veggies in the bowl and mix together well.

Nutrition: Calories 145, 9 grams carbs, 4 grams protein, 7.5 grams fat

32. Greek Spaghetti Squash

Prep twenty min/serves two

Ingredients:

Feta cheese, crumbles, two tablespoons

Salt, .25 teaspoon

Baby spinach, torn, one cup

Baked spaghetti squash, two cups

Cherry tomatoes, six cuts in half

Thyme, fresh, chopped, one teaspoon

Chickpeas, .3 cup, rinse and drain

Garlic, minced, one teaspoon

Red onion, thin slice, .25 cup

Olive oil, two tablespoons

Cook the garlic and the onion in the olive oil for five minutes. Add in the tomatoes, thyme, and chickpeas and cook three more minutes. Add in the salt, spinach, and spaghetti squash and cook five minutes stirring constantly. Sprinkle on the feta cheese all over the top and serve.

Nutrition: Calories 272, 14 grams carbs, 11 grams protein, 10 grams fat

33. Tomato, Squash, and Red Pepper Gratin

Prep thirty min/cook one and one-half hour/serve six

Ingredients:

Beefsteak tomato, one large, cut into eight slices

Olive oil, two tablespoons

Gruyere cheese, .75 cup

Heavy cream, .5 cup

Black pepper, one teaspoon

Salt, .25 teaspoon and .25 teaspoon

Thyme, fresh, chopped, two teaspoons

Basil, fresh, .25 cup

Garlic, minced, one tablespoon

Yellow squash, one pound, cut into quarter inch thick slices

Red bell pepper, chopped, one and one half cup

Red onion, chopped, two cups

Olive oil, five teaspoons divided

Heat oven to 375. Cook garlic, squash, bell pepper, and onion for five minutes in four teaspoons of the olive oil. Stir in the pepper, salt, thyme, and basil. Mix together in a medium-sized mixing bowl the cheese, cream, and salt until they are well blended. Pour this mix over the vegetables and place the entire mix into a nine by thirteen baking pan. Lay the tomatoes over the top of the veggie mixture and bake for forty-five minutes. Use the remaining basil to sprinkle on top and serve.

Nutrition: Calories 235, 17 grams carbs, 13 grams protein, 12 grams fat

34. Cheesy Cauliflower Soup

Prep ten min/cook twenty min/serves six

Ingredients:

Cheddar cheese, grated, eight ounces

Heavy cream, two cups

Vegetable stock, two cups

Cauliflower, grated, one large head

Black pepper, one teaspoon

Salt, .5 teaspoon

Shallot, one

Garlic, two cloves minced

Olive oil, one tablespoon

Cook the shallot and the garlic in a large pot with the olive oil. Place the cauliflower in the pot and mix well with the olive oil and cook for five minutes. Add in the heavy cream and the vegetable stock and bring the mixture to a boil. Turn the heat back down and simmer this mixture for five minutes. Take the pot off the heat and add in the pepper, salt, and cheese, stirring gently for one minute and serve.

Nutrition: Calories 227, 9 grams carbs, 10 grams protein, 16 grams fat

35. Stuffed Artichokes

Prep forty five min/cook thirty min/serves six

Ingredients:

Artichokes, three

Cottage cheese, .5 cup

Celery salt, .25 teaspoon

Mushroom, chopped, .5 cup

Salt, one teaspoon

Onion, minced, two tablespoons

Lemon juice, two tablespoons

Egg, one slightly beat

Parsley, chopped, one tablespoon

Chili sauce, one tablespoon

Heat oven to 375. Tear off and discard the outside leaves of the artichokes. Cut the inside in half across the middle. Drop the halves into boiling water and cook for twenty minutes. Mix together the cottage cheese, onions, egg, mushrooms, lemon juice, chili sauce, seasonings, and parsley and spoon this mixture into the boiled artichoke hearts. Place the filled hearts into a baking pan and bake for thirty minutes.

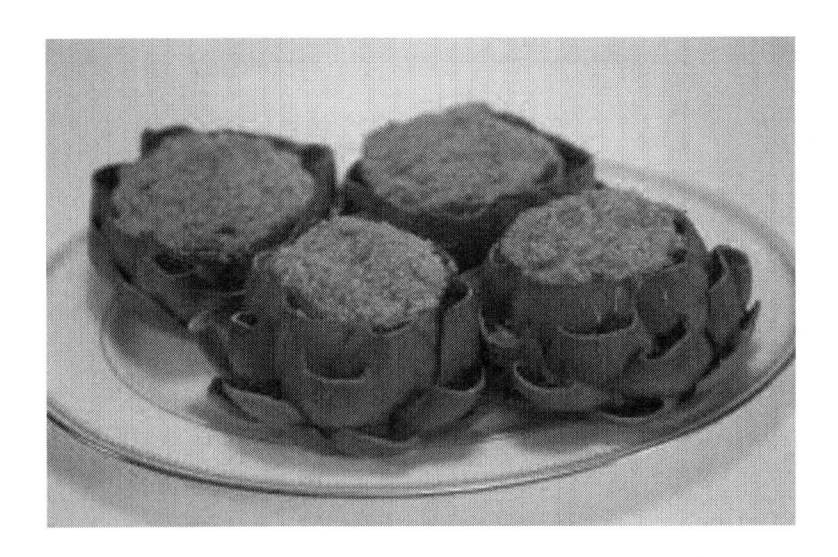

Nutrition: Calories 425, 17 grams carbs, 18 grams protein, 21 grams fat

36. Lima Bean Casserole

Prep fifteen min/cook thirty min/serves five

Ingredients:
Lima beans, canned two cups
Cheese, mild cheddar, shredded, one half cup
Butter, one tablespoon
Dry mustard, two teaspoons
Salt, one teaspoon
Black pepper, one teaspoon
Lemon juice, two teaspoons

Heat oven to 375. Drain the beans and save the liquid. Dump the drained beans into an eight by eight baking pan. Add bean liquid and butter to a skillet and heat until the butter melts. Add in the salt, pepper, dry mustard, and lemon juice and stir together well. Pour this mix over the beans in the baking pan and cover with the shredded cheese. Bake for thirty minutes.

Nutrition: Calories 194, 19 grams carbs, 6 grams protein, 7 grams fat

37. Kale and Chickpea Salad with Poppy seed Lemon Dressing

Prep thirty min/serves four

Ingredients:

POPPYSEED LEMON DRESSING

Poppy seeds, .25 teaspoon

Lemon juice, one tablespoon

Dijon mustard, one tablespoon

Olive oil, one tablespoon

KALE

Chickpeas, one cup

Kale, four cups washed, remove stems

Olive oil, two tablespoons

Salt, one teaspoon

Black pepper, two teaspoons

Heat oven to 325. Lay kale out on a cookie sheet, drizzle with olive oil and bake for ten minutes. Mix all of the ingredients that are listed for the dressing and blend them well. Cook the chickpeas in olive oil for fifteen minutes, stirring often. Take the baked kale from the oven and place it in a medium sized mixing bowl. Pour the chickpeas and the dressing onto the kale and toss all ingredients gently until they are well mixed.

Nutrition: Calories 334, 15 grams carbs, 4 grams protein, 26 grams fat

38. Eggplant Casserole

Prep fifteen min/cook thirty min/serves six

Ingredients:
Cheese, grated, .75 cup
Eggplant, one medium
Tomato soup, one can
Onion, chopped, .25 cup
Olive oil, two tablespoons

Heat oven to 375. Peel the eggplant and dice it into bite-sized cubes. Drop the cubes into water that is boiling and cook for five minutes, then drain well. Put the eggplant in a nine by nine baking pan. Fry the onion in the olive oil for five minutes. Pour in the soup and the cheese and cook, stirring often, until the cheese is melted. Pout this mixture over the eggplant and bake for thirty minutes.

Nutrition: Calories 267, 19 grams carbs, 13 grams protein, 9 grams fat

39. Butternut Squash with Mustard Vinaigrette

Prep twenty min/cook fifty min/serves six

Ingredients:
Squash, three small butternuts peeled, seeded and cut in half
Shallots, eight, cut into wedges
Dry mustard, one tablespoon
Olive oil, four tablespoons
Salt, .5 teaspoon
Black pepper, one teaspoon
Rice wine vinegar, one tablespoon
Parsley, chopped, .25 cup

Heat oven to 375. Use a large mixing bowl to mix the squash and the shallots with the pepper, salt, and olive oil, tossing to mix well and coat all pieces. Arrange the squash and shallots on a cookie sheet and bake for fifty minutes. While the veggies are baking make vinaigrette with the rice wine vinegar, dry mustard, and the parsley. Arrange the baked veggies on a serving dish and drizzle the vinaigrette over them and serve.

Nutrition: Calories 135, 11 grams carbs, 1 gram protein, 10 grams fat

40. Corn and Okra Casserole

Prep twenty min/cook thirty min/serves six

Ingredients:

Okra, one pound

Butter, three tablespoons

Tomatoes, two large diced

Corn, whole kernel, one can

Onion, one small, sliced

Green bell pepper, one cleaned and sliced

Garlic, one clove sliced

Parsley, chopped, one tablespoon

Heat oven to 375. Cut the okra into bite-sized chunks. Cook the okra, onion, garlic, and green pepper in the butter for ten minutes. Stir in the tomatoes and the parsley and cook an additional ten minutes. Pour in the corn and dump the entire mixture into a nine by nine baking pan and bake, not covered, for thirty minutes.

Nutrition: Calories 125, 17 grams carbs, 4 grams protein, 2 grams fat

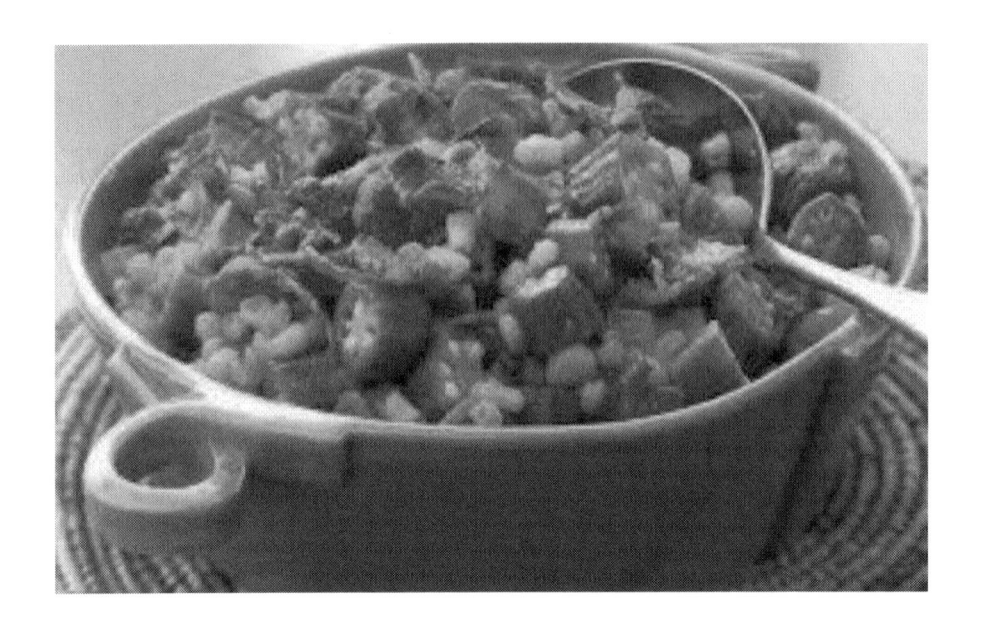

Chapter 8: Keto Sauces

When cooking any kind of food the secret to the success or failure of the dish often lies in the sauce that is covering the food. And think how many times a particular sauce has made a good dish taste even better. Salads and vegetables can sometimes be boring, but with a good sauce to drizzle over they suddenly become flavorful and exciting. And life would not be complete without a wonderful cheese sauce to pour on just about everything.

But too often keto dieters are left out in the cold because the sauces that are ready made in the grocery store contain many starches and sugars that just do not fit into the keto diet. So here is assembled some recipes for sauces that are keto friendly and will help flavor your new path to healthiness.

1. Avocado Cilantro Sauce

Prep four min/cook one min

This is a great dressing for any dish with a Mexican flair like Huevos Rancheros. It is also great when used as a dressing on any salad or a bowl of mixed garden veggies.

Ingredients:

MCT oil, two tablespoons*

Cilantro, fresh, three bunches

Lemon juice, two tablespoons

Lime juice, two tablespoons

Garlic, cloves, two

Salt, .5 teaspoon

Water, .5 cup

Place the liquid ingredients except for the water in a food processor or a blender and mix together. Then add in the dry ingredients and mix well until the sauce is creamy and smooth. Add the water by the teaspoon if it is needed to make the sauce less thick. This sauce is best used immediately but can also be stored in the refrigerator for no more than three days.

Nutrition per one quarter cup: Calories 109, 2.7 grams carbs, 2.8 grams protein, 8.9 grams fat

MCT oil is a fat supplement that can be added to foods to make them mix more smoothly and provide a higher fat content. They are easy to digest and have many health benefits for the keto dieter.

2. Pesto Sauce

Prep five min/cook five min/

Pesto sauce can be used as a dip for celery and cucumber sticks, a topping for baked cheese like Brie, or a sauce for cauliflower rice.

Ingredients:

Salt, .5 teaspoon

Black pepper, one teaspoon

Butter, two tablespoons

Garlic, cloves, two

MCT oil, .5 cup

Basil, fresh leaves, two cups

Mix together in a blender or a food processor the garlic, MCT oil, and basil until completely combined. Then add the butter and the parmesan. This is best used immediately. It can be kept stored for up to a week by keeping it in an airtight container in the refrigerator. Before sealing the lid pour a thin layer of olive oil over the pesto to help keep air out. This can be poured off or stirred in when you want to use it again.

Nutrition per one-third cup: Calories 323, 4 grams carbs, 7 grams protein, 32 grams fat

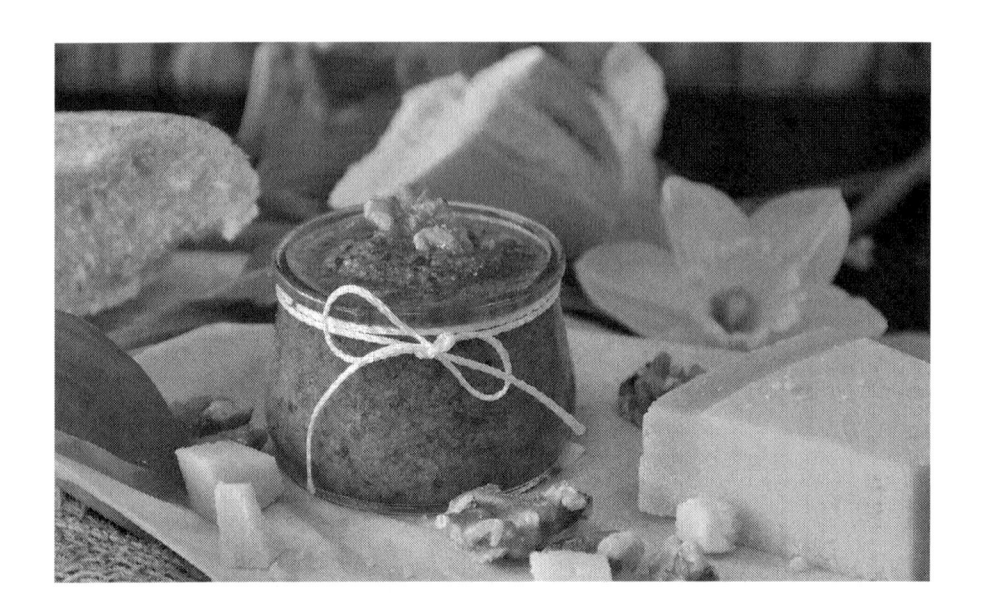

3. Mustard Sauce

Prep five min/cook twelve hours

Ingredients:

Turmeric, two teaspoons

Salt, two teaspoon

Apple cider vinegar, five tablespoons

Water, one cup

Mustard seed powder, four ounces

Mustard seeds, four ounces

Use a spice grinder or a pestle and mortar to grind coarsely the whole mustard seeds. In a bowl for mixing combine the ground seeds with the turmeric powder, mustard powder, and salt. When they are well mixed add the water and blend until the mix is very smooth. Let the mixture sit for ten minutes. Then mix in the apple cider vinegar. Scoop the mustard into a glass bowl or a glass jar. Then the dressing will need to stay covered in the refrigerator for a minimum of ten hours before using. This mustard will stay good for up to a year if kept refrigerated.

Nutrition per one tablespoon: Calories 3, .3 grams carbs, .2 grams protein, .2 grams fat

4. Lemon Herb Sauce

Prep fifteen min

Ingredients:

Red pepper flakes, one teaspoon

Black pepper, two teaspoons

Salt, one teaspoon

Olive oil, .25 cup

Lemon juice, two tablespoons

Lemon zest, two tablespoons

Cilantro, one bunch chopped

Mint, one bunch chopped

Parsley, one bunch chopped

Garlic, clove, one peel, and smash

Shallot, one, peel, and chop

Place the lemon zest, herbs, garlic, and shallot in a blender or a food processor and combine. Pour in the olive oil and the lemon juice and blend into a smooth sauce. Add in the red pepper flakes, black pepper, and the salt and mix one last time. This sauce will keep for no more than one week.

Nutrition per quarter cup: Calories 195, 12 grams carbs, 1 gram protein, 15 grams fat

5. Creamy Alfredo

Prep five min/cook ten min

Paired with zucchini noodles this makes a great pasta style dish that are keto friendly.

Ingredients:

Salt, 5 teaspoon

Nutmeg, ground, .25 teaspoon

White pepper, .25 teaspoon

Egg, one

Butter, two tablespoons at room temperature

Parmesan cheese, fresh grated, two ounces

Cream cheese, three ounces at room temperature

Heavy cream, one cup

Slowly over low heat melt the cream cheese and the butter together. Stir often to mix well. Pour in one-quarter cup of the heavy cream and raise the heat slightly, stirring often until the cream is well mixed and the mixture is hot. Stir in one-fourth of the Parmesan cheese and stir frequently until it is melted. Take turns adding in the heavy cream and the Parmesan cheese until both have been completely added. Crack the egg and drop it into a bowl and beat it to mix it well. When the cream and the cheese have been added and the sauce is hot pour in the egg while continuously stirring the sauce. Continue to cook the sauce and lower the heat while stirring frequently for about two to three minutes until the sauce begins to become thick. Add in the seasonings and stir well and serve.

Nutrition per quarter cup: Calories 410, 3 grams carbs, 9 grams protein, 41 grams fat

6. Marinara Sauce

Prep five min/cook ten min
Also great to use with any dish with an Italian flavor such as pairing it with zucchini noodles to make keto friendly spaghetti. This would also be good with Eggplant Parmesan.
Ingredients:
Parsley, fine chop, two tablespoons

Red Wine Vinegar, one tablespoon

Black pepper, one teaspoon

Salt, one teaspoon

Tomato puree, three cups

Oregano, fine chop, two teaspoons

Thyme, fine chop, two teaspoons

Onion flakes, two teaspoons

Garlic, one clove

Olive oil, two tablespoons

Put the oregano, thyme, onion flakes, garlic, and olive oil in a pot and mix well. Pour the tomato puree in and mix it with the seasonings until smooth. Set the heat on the stove on low and stir in the salt, pepper, and the red wine vinegar and then bring the mixture to simmer. Remove the pot from the heat and thoroughly mix in the parsley.

Nutrition per half cup: Calories 27, 2 grams carbs, .5 grams protein, 2 grams fat

7. White Cheese Sauce

Prep five min/cook twenty min

This sauce is great when served on any hot vegetable, particularly on asparagus or green beans.

Ingredients:

Mozzarella cheese, shredded, two cups

Heavy cream, one cup

Butter, one cup

Cream cheese, eight ounces

Combine the heavy cream, butter, and the cream cheese in a pot and set it over low heat. As the ingredients begin to soften and melt stir constantly to prevent sticking or burning. When all of these ingredients have become liquid and are well mixed together then add in the mozzarella cheese. Continue stirring constantly until the cheese is fully melted and well mixed in. This will keep for no more than three days and just needs rewarming over low heat to use later.

Nutrition per half cup: Calories 389, 2 grams carbs, 6 grams protein, 39 grams fat

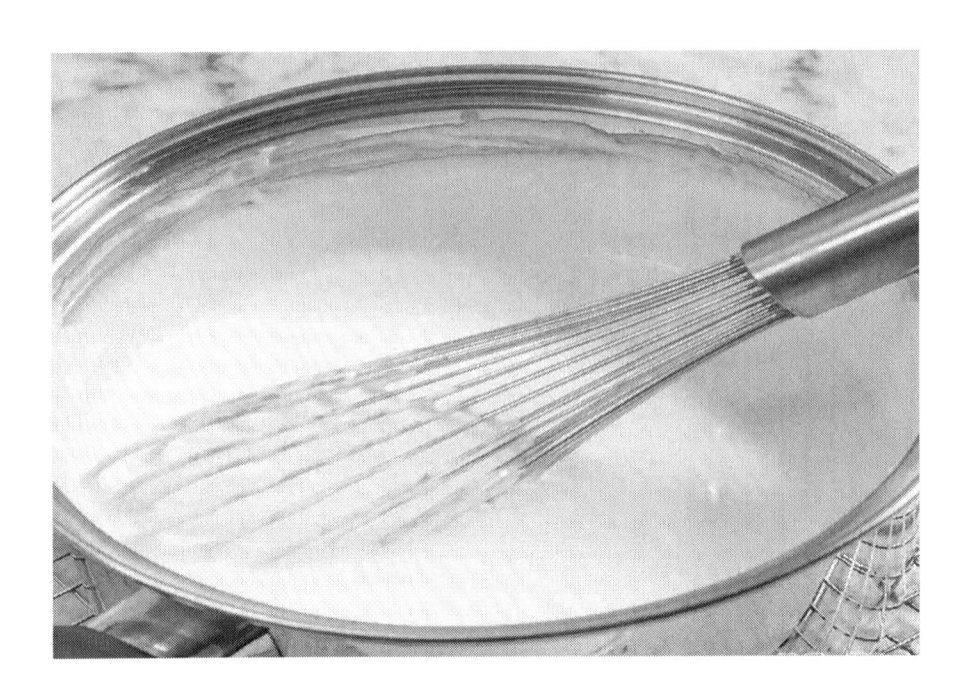

8. Sweet Soy Sauce

Prep five min/cook twenty min

This is a must-have sauce for any Asian inspired dish, particularly cauliflower fried rice!

Tamari sauce, one cup

Xylitol, one and one quarter cup

Place both ingredients in a pot and turn the heat on to a low setting, stirring often. Cook this over the low heat for about twenty minutes or until the xylitol has completely dissolved and the sauce has become slightly thick. This sauce will keep for up to three weeks when stored in an airtight container in the refrigerator.

Nutrition per one tablespoon: Calories 8, 1 gram carbs, 2 grams protein, 0 grams fat

9. Pepper Sauce

Prep five min/cook fifteen min

This is a great sauce to use to flavor any type of cooked vegetables.

Ingredients:

Salt, .5 teaspoon

Xanthan gum*, .5 teaspoon

White pepper, ground, .25 teaspoon

Black pepper, .5 teaspoon

Green peppercorns, two tablespoons

Heavy cream, .5 cup

Vegetable broth, one cup

Yellow onion, one-half medium, diced fine

Butter, one tablespoon

In a pot fry the onion in the butter using high heat for five minutes. Pour in the vegetable broth and mix well. Stir in the green peppercorns, black pepper, and white pepper with the heavy cream and let this simmer for seven to eight minutes while stirring constantly. Add in the salt and the xanthan gum and stir well and then remove the pot from the heat.

*Xanthan gum is an ingredient used to thicken soups and sauces, much like cornstarch is. However, it is much more keto friendly. A tablespoon of cornstarch has 117 grams of carbs where a tablespoon of xanthan gum has only 2 grams of carbs.

Nutrition per quarter cup: Calories 144, 3 grams carbs, 2 grams protein, 8 grams fat

10. Whole Egg Mayonnaise

Prep fifteen min/cook one min

This mayonnaise recipe is keto friendly and guaranteed gluten free if that is a concern for you. It can be used as the mayonnaise ingredient in recipes and also to make an amazing egg salad.

Ingredients:

White vinegar, one tablespoon

Black pepper, .25 teaspoon

Salt, .25 teaspoon

Olive oil, twenty ounces

Sesame oil, seven ounces

Dijon mustard, two tablespoons

Eggs, two large

Drop the eggs and the mustard into a blender or a food processor and mix together on medium speed for three minutes. Mix the two oils together and slowly pour this liquid into the blender or food processor while it is running on a slow speed. If you mix the oil in too quickly it will separate and not become mayonnaise. After all of the oil is mixed in the mix in the pepper and salt and mix for one more minute. You may add the vinegar if the mixture seems to be too thick.

Nutrition per one quarter cup: Calories 164, .1 gram carbs, .3 grams protein, 18 grams fat

11. Guacamole

Prep five min/cook one min

A must have for any Mexican inspired dish.

Ingredients:

Sour cream, full fat, one tablespoon

Scallions, thin sliced, two tablespoons

Cilantro, finely chopped, one tablespoon

Paprika, .25 teaspoon

Chili powder, .25 teaspoon

Garlic, minced, one tablespoon

Cumin, .25 teaspoon

Black pepper, .25 teaspoon

Salt, .25 teaspoon

Lime juice, one tablespoon

Avocado, one medium

Carefully slice open the avocado and take out the seed. Remove the peel and put the avocado into a bowl with the lime juice and then mash it well. Stir in the remaining ingredients until the guacamole is well mixed.

Nutrition per quarter cup: Calories 115, 7 grams carbs, 2 grams protein, 10 grams fat

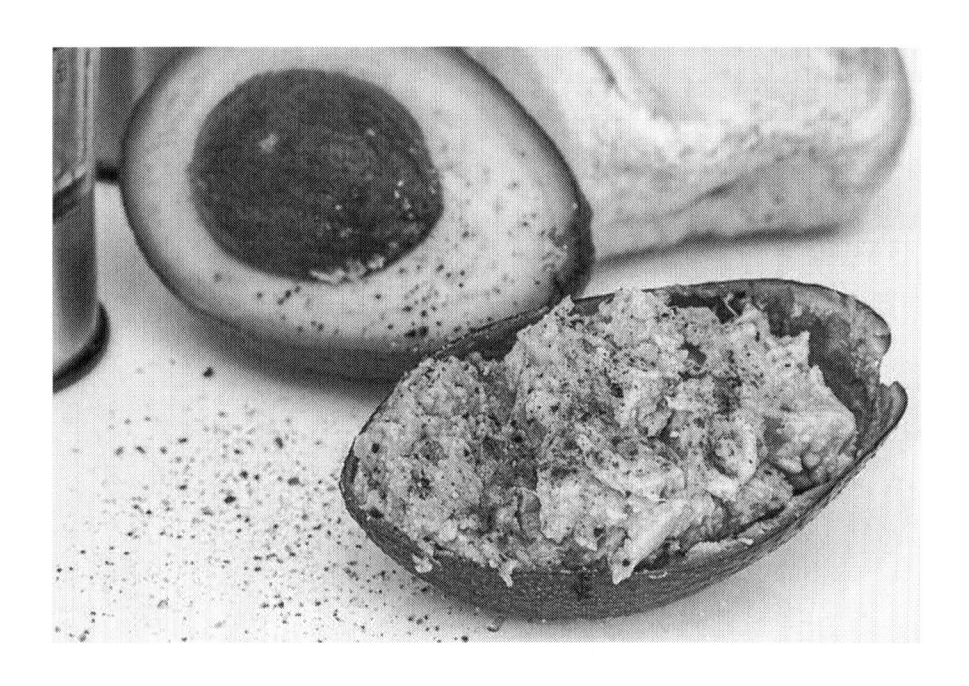

12. Avocado Garlic Caesar Dressing

Prep five min

Romaine lettuce might become your new best friend.

Ingredients:

Lemon juice, one tablespoon

Dijon mustard, two teaspoons

Parmesan cheese, shredded, .5 cup

Anchovy paste, .5 teaspoon

Garlic, cloves, two chopped fine

Worcestershire sauce, one teaspoon

Avocado, one medium size peeled and mashed

Mayonnaise, one cup

Use a medium sized mixing bowl to put all of the ingredients in and combine well until the mixture is smooth. Keep the dressing in an airtight container in the refrigerator for no more than one week.

Nutrition per quarter cup: Calories 74, 2.3 grams carbs, 2.2 grams protein, 6 grams fat

13. Lemon Curd

Prep ten min/cook ten min

This is the perfect topping for keto friendly cake or custard or simply with a bowl of low carb berries.

Ingredients:

Egg yolk, one

Eggs, three whole

Butter, one half cup

Xylitol, .5 cup

Lemons, four whole for zest and juice

Using the top of the double boiler* place the butter, xylitol, and zest the lemons and squeeze all of the juice out. The bottom part of the double boiler should have simmering water in it as the pan is sitting over low heat. Blend together the egg yolk and the eggs and then mix this gently into the warm mixture. Cook this mix while stirring often for ten minutes. This mix will store for up to two weeks in the refrigerator.

If you do not own a double boiler you can set a smaller pan or heat-proof bowl over a larger pot.

Nutrition per half cup: Calories 258, 2 grams carbs, 7 grams protein, 25 grams fat

14. Ranch Dressing

Prep ten min

Ingredients:

Black pepper, .5 teaspoon

Salt, .5 teaspoon

Dill, fresh, fine chop, one teaspoon

Chives, fresh, fine chop, one tablespoon

Parsley, fresh, fine chop, one tablespoon

Onion powder, .5 teaspoon

Garlic powder, two tablespoons

Coconut cream, .25 cup

Mayonnaise, .25 cup

Use a medium size mixing bowl to put all of the ingredients in and mix gently until all of the ingredients for the dressing are well mixed. This ranch dressing will keep very well in the refrigerator for up to four days if tightly covered.

Nutrition per one quarter cup: Calories 66, 1 gram carbs, 0 grams protein, 8 grams fat

15. Italian Dressing

Prep five min

Ingredients:

Olive oil, .75 cup

Red wine vinegar, .25 cup

Black pepper, .25 teaspoon

Salt, .5 teaspoon

Garlic, minced, one tablespoon

Oregano, dried, one teaspoon

Parsley, fresh chop, one tablespoon

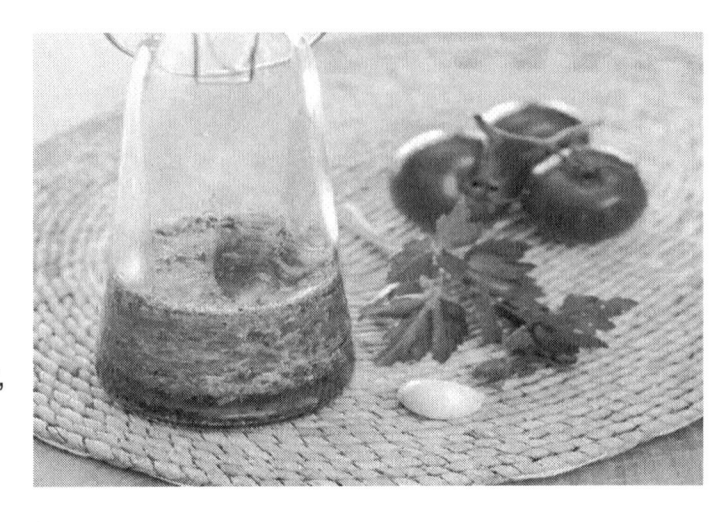

Use a medium sized mixing bowl to put all of the ingredients into and mix well until all of the ingredients for the dressing are blended well. This is a good dressing to store in an airtight jar in the refrigerator for up to four days.

Nutrition per one quarter cup: Calories 91, 1 gram carbs, 0 grams protein, 10 grams fat

Chapter 9: Keto Desserts

No proper meal plan would be worth anything if it did not leave room for dessert. After all, we are human, and sometimes humans just need something sweet at the end of the day. The problem has always been finding desserts that satisfy the sweet tooth without adding sugar to the diet. Here are some delicious keto friendly desserts guaranteed to please even the most finicky eater.

1. Cheesecake Keto Fat Bombs

Prep ten minutes
Ingredients:
Dark chocolate chips, mini size, .5 cup
Xylitol, two tablespoons
Peanut butter, creamy, .25 cup
Cream cheese, four ounces, softened to room temperature

Cream together the xylitol, cream cheese, and peanut butter until all ingredients are mixed well and the mixture is smooth. Use a tablespoon to form small balls about an inch across in measurement and roll them in the chocolate chips. Lay the fat bombs out on a plate covered with wax paper or parchment paper and set them in the freezer for two hours. When the bombs are frozen then place them into a bowl with a lid and keep them stored in the refrigerator.

Nutrition per bomb: Calories 93, 1.3 grams carbs, 1.2 grams protein, 9.7 grams fat

2. Cinnamon Sugar Donuts

Prep ten minutes/cook fifteen min

Ingredients:

DONUTS

Baking soda, .5 teaspoon

Baking powder, one and one half teaspoons

Cinnamon, ground, one teaspoon

Xanthan gum, .25 teaspoon

Coconut flour, .5 tablespoon

Almond flour, one cup

Xylitol, .25 cup

Butter or ghee, two tablespoons

Vanilla extract, one teaspoon

Apple cider vinegar, .25 teaspoon

Almond milk, .25 cup

Eggs, two large at room temperature

TOPPING

Cinnamon sugar coating:

Butter, one and one half tablespoon

Cinnamon, ground, one teaspoon

Xylitol, .25 cup

Chocolate glaze:

Xylitol, one teaspoon

Coconut oil, one teaspoon melted

Dark chocolate, sugar-free, two ounces melted

Heat oven to 350. Cream together the xylitol, butter, vanilla extract, apple cider vinegar, almond milk, and the eggs until this mixture is smooth and well blended. Use another bowl to mix together the salt, baking soda, baking powder, cinnamon, xanthan gum, coconut flour, and the almond flour until well blended. Combine the dry ingredients with the wet ingredients in small amounts until both are well mixed. Drop the batter in equal amounts into a mini donut pan or a muffin pan only filling the wells to three fourths full. Bake the donuts for twelve to fifteen minutes for the mini donuts or twenty-one to twenty-four minutes for the regular sized ones. When the donuts have cooled slightly use either the cinnamon sugar topping or the chocolate glaze to top them with and serve immediately.

Nutrition per donut: Calories 86, 2 grams carbs, 2 grams protein, 8 grams fat

3. One Minute Brownie

Prep two min/cook one min

Ingredients:

Chocolate chunks, one tablespoon

Almond milk, .25 cup

Egg, one

Cocoa powder, one tablespoon

Baking powder, .5 teaspoon

Stevia, one tablespoon

Coconut flour, one tablespoon

Chocolate protein powder, one scoop

Use lard to lightly grease an oven-safe ramekin or a microwave safe bowl. Mix together completely all of the dry ingredients in a small bowl. Add the chocolate chunks, milk, and egg and mix well until the ingredients have formed a smooth batter. If you decide to cook this in the oven then bake it at 350 for fifteen minutes. If you are using the microwave then cook it for one minute.

Nutrition: Calories 129, 3 grams carbs, 3 grams protein, 4 grams fat

4. Peanut Butter Balls

Prep twenty min

Ingredients:

Chocolate chips, sugar-free, eight ounces

Powdered sweetener, one cup

Peanut butter, one cup

Peanuts, salted, one cup chopped finely

Use a medium-sized bowl to cream together the sweetener, peanut butter, and the chopped peanuts until mixed very well. Separate the dough into eighteen equal size pieces and roll into the shape of a ball. Put the balls not touching on a cookie sheet and put them in the refrigerator until they are cold for about one hour. After one hour melt the chocolate chips in the microwave until they are completely melted. Then dip the chilled peanut butter balls into the melted chocolate one at a time until all of them are well coated. Place the chocolate coated balls back on to the cookie sheet and refrigerate until the chocolate sets.

Nutrition per peanut butter ball: Calories 194, 4 grams carbs, 7 grams protein, 17 grams fat

5. Cinnamon Roll Cheesecake

Prep twenty min/cook thirty min

Ingredients:

CRUST

Butter, two tablespoons melted

Cinnamon, .5 teaspoon

Sugar-free sweetener, two tablespoons

Almond flour, .5 cup

CHEESECAKE FILLING

Cinnamon, two teaspoons

Egg, one large

Vanilla extract, .5 teaspoon

Sour cream, .25 cup

Sugar-free sweetener, five tablespoons divided

Cream cheese, six ounces softened to room temperature

FROSTING

Heavy cream, two tablespoons

Vanilla extract, .25 teaspoon

Sugar-free confectioners' sugar, three tablespoons

Butter, one tablespoon softened to room temperature

Heat oven to 325. Use paper cups to place in six holes of a muffin pan. Cream together three tablespoons of the sweetener and the cream cheese. Then blend in the egg, vanilla, and sour cream until all ingredients are well mixed. In a separate small bowl mix well the cinnamon and the leftover two tablespoons of the sweetener. Use a spoon to drop three-fourths of a teaspoon of the cream cheese mixture into each of the six muffin papers. Then use a bit of the cinnamon sugar mix to sprinkle on top. Repeat this process two times more until all of the batter and all of the sugar-cinnamon mixture are used up. Bake for seventeen minutes and then let the cheesecakes cool for thirty minutes before placing them into the refrigerator at least for two hours. While the cheesecakes are chilling mix the frosting ingredients and then dribble the frosting over the cheesecakes.

Nutrition per cheesecake: Calories 237, 3 grams carbs, 5 grams protein, 21 grams fat

6. Brownies

Prep ten min/cook twenty min
Ingredients:
Vanilla extract, .5 teaspoon
Eggs, three at room temperature
Dark chocolate, two ounces
Butter, ten tablespoon
Baking powder, .5 teaspoon
Xylitol, .75 cup

Cocoa powder, .25 cup

Almond flour, .5 cup

Heat oven to 350. Use lard or butter to grease an eight by eight baking pan. Mix completely together all of the dry ingredients until the mix is smooth and has no lumps. Melt carefully the chocolate and the butter together in the microwave for one minute or until they are melted together. Whisk in the dry ingredients by gently folding the wet into the dry just until the ingredients are mixed. Spoon the batter into the baking pan and use the back of the spoon to smooth the batter evenly in the pan. Bake the brownies for twenty-five minutes and let the brownies cool for at least two hours before cutting them.

Nutrition per two inches by two-inch brownie: Calories 116, 2 grams carbs, 2 grams proteins, 11 grams fat

7. No Churn Ice Cream

Prep five minutes/cook thirty minutes

Ingredients:

MCT oil, .5 cup

Vanilla extract, one teaspoon

Xylitol, .3 cup

Heavy cream, three cups divided into two cups and one cup
Butter, three tablespoons

Set a large pan on the stove over medium heat to melt the butter. Add in the two cups of the heavy cream and the xylitol. Mix this well and bring the mix to a boil and then lower the heat and allow the mix to simmer gently. Keep simmering this mix for thirty to forty-five minutes while you stir it occasionally until the mix becomes thick. Dump this mixture into a large bowl and let it cool until it has reached room temperature. When the mixture in the bowl has reached room temperature stir in the vanilla extract and the MCT oil. Use a whisk or a hand mixer to beat the leftover cup of heavy cream until it forms stiff peaks when the mixer is lifted out. Gradually and very gently fold the beaten cream into the larger mix in the other bowl. Quickly put the mixture into a bowl that is safe for the freezer and place it in the freezer for six hours.

Nutrition per one-half cup: Calories 345, 2 grams carbs, 2 grams protein, 36 grams fat

8. White Chocolate Peanut Butter Blondies

Prep ten minutes/cook twenty-five minutes
Ingredients:
Raw cocoa butter, .25 cup
Sweetener, .25 cup

Coconut flour, one tablespoon

Almond flour, .25 cup

Melted raw cocoa butter, three tablespoons

Vanilla extract, one teaspoon

Eggs, two

Butter, softened, four tablespoons

Peanut butter, .5 cup

Heat oven to 350. Use lard or butter to grease a nine by nine baking pan. Combine the melted raw cocoa butter, vanilla extract, eggs, butter, and the peanut butter until smooth and creamy. Stir in the chopped cocoa butter, sweetener, and the two flours. As soon as all of the ingredients listed are well mixed then spoon the mixture into the greased pan and use the spoon to smooth the batter in the pan. Bake the blondies for twenty-five minutes and let them cool for at least two hours before you cut them

Nutrition per one piece two and one quarter by two and one quarter: Calories 103, 1 gram carbs, 3 grams protein, 9 grams fat

9. Chocolate Chip Cookies

Prep fifteen min/ cook fifteen min

Ingredients:

Dark chocolate chips, .75 cup

Sugar substitute, .25 cup

Salt, .25 teaspoon

Almond four, two and three fourth cups

Vanilla extract, two teaspoon

Heavy cream, two tablespoons

Butter, .5 cup (one stick) melted

Eggs, two large

Heat the oven to 350. Cream together the vanilla, heavy cream, butter, and the eggs until it forms a smooth batter. Blend in the sweetener, salt, and the almond flour. Gently fold the dark chocolate chips into the mixed batter. Make the batter into one inch balls using a spoon and set the balls about three inches apart on a cookie sheet. Use the bottom of a lightly greased glass to flatten the balls about halfway. Bake each batch of cookies for sixteen to nineteen minutes and let cool.

Nutrition per one cookie: Calories 96, 3 grams carbs, 2 grams protein, 9 grams fat

10. Chocolate Frosty

Prep ten min/freeze forty-five minutes

Ingredients:

Salt, .18 teaspoon

Vanilla extract, one teaspoon

Powdered sugar sweetener, keto friendly, three tablespoons

Cocoa powder, unsweetened, two tablespoons

Heavy whipping cream, one and one half cup

Using the whisk on a stand mixer or using a hand mixer, cream together the salt, vanilla, sweetener, cocoa, and the heavy cream until the mixture forms stiff peaks when the beater blade is removed from the mix. Freeze for forty-five minutes and serve.

Nutrition per one fourth: Calories 241, 4 grams carbs, 3 grams protein, 25 grams fat

Chapter 10: Two Week Meal Plan

This is a sample two week meal plan of what menus might look like for the first two weeks of your keto diet plan. All of these recipes can be found in this book. This is only a suggestion of what your daily meals might look like. Feel free to change meals around or even come up with some of your own. The more you experiment the more this diet will be truly your own.

Day 1

Breakfast	Maple Oatmeal
Lunch	Grilled Eggplant Rollups
Dinner	Cauliflower Rice with Mushroom Risotto

Day 2

Breakfast	Egg Breakfast Muffins
Lunch	Greek Fattoush Salad
Dinner	Eggplant Chickpea Stew

Day 3

Breakfast	Tomato Omelet
Lunch	Herb and Halloumi Tomato Salad
Dinner	Zucchini Soup

Day 4

Breakfast	Banana Pancakes
Lunch	Nicoise Salad
Dinner	Spicy Lentil Soup

Day 5

Breakfast	Chia Breakfast Pudding
Lunch	Greek Collar Wraps
Dinner	Fried Goat Cheese with Charred Veggies

Day 6

Breakfast	Peppers and Onions Scrambled Eggs
Lunch	Sprout Wraps
Dinner	Cauliflower Fried Rice

Day 7

Breakfast	Huevos Rancheros
Lunch	Vegetarian Club Salad
Dinner	Mediterranean Pasta

Day 8

Breakfast	Baked Italian Skillet Eggs
Lunch	Chickpea Salad
Dinner	Zucchini and Spinach Lasagna

Day 9

Breakfast	Vegetable Quiche
Lunch	Cheesy Cauliflower Soup
Dinner	Spiral Zucchini and Grape Tomatoes

Day 10

Breakfast	Punjabi Egg Curry
Lunch	Eggplant Casserole
Dinner	Tuscany Vegetable Soup

Day 11

Breakfast	Baked Avocado Egg
Lunch	Lima Bean Casserole
Dinner	Tomato Squash and Red Pepper Gratin

Day 12

Breakfast	Mushroom Sandwich with Eggs and Greens
Lunch	Corn and Okra Casserole
Dinner	Butternut Squash with Mustard Vinaigrette

Day 13

Breakfast	Curried Tofu Scramble
Lunch	Roast Baby Eggplant
Dinner	Cheese and Broccoli Cauliflower Rice

Day 14

Breakfast	Cream Cheese Pancakes
Lunch	Stuffed Artichokes
Dinner	Squash and Sweet Potato Patties

Chapter 11: Making the Keto Diet Your Own

Now that you have the recipes, the shopping list, and the little extras that are contained in this book you are ready to begin your journey into the world of keto dieting and better overall health. Deciding to begin the keto diet is not quite like beginning any other diet plan you may have ever tried before. As you have probably noticed doing the keto diet properly will require a bit more work than doing any other diet. The keto diet requires meal planning and creative thinking. You may want to cook a week's worth of meals at one time and freeze them in serving portions for later. You might find that you can't eat all of that fresh food before it spoils and you begin to rely more on canned or frozen food, but that is okay. If you really want to eat only fresh foods it may require more frequent visits to the grocery store, and that is totally your decision. However you make the keto diet work for you is the right way, because this is your diet.

You cannot avoid ketosis if you truly want to succeed on the keto diet. Remember that the process of ketosis is the process by which your body begins to get rid of all that excess fat that you are carrying around. When you begin to go into the state of ketosis you may think you have the flu, because the symptoms are very similar. You may feel irritable, lethargic, and you might vomit or have diarrhea. Unfortunately, these symptoms can last for up to a week but once you enter ketosis you will remain there as long as you continuously restrict your carbohydrate intake. If you suddenly increase your carb intake your body will come out of ketosis and you will not continue to burn fat as you did before. In fact, you might even gain a few pounds. And if you begin to restrict your carbs again you will go through ketosis again. This is why keto is not considered to be a diet as much as it is considered to be a lifestyle choice.

People will tell you that you cannot live without carbohydrates and that your brain needs the fuel from sugar to function completely, and this is just not true. When your body no longer has incoming carbs from food consumption to burn for fuel it will turn to its stored fat deposits for energy sources. This is exactly what you want to happen, as this is how you will begin to lose weight. And your brain will survive just fine on the ketones that are produced during ketosis. Just remember not to exceed your protein intake on a regular basis because your body will turn the excess protein into blood sugar and this can also throw your body out of ketosis.

This is how our bodies were made to function when the first human was made centuries ago. The human body is a very efficient, smooth running machine. As long as we do not interfere with our body's processes too much then it will continue to work at its peak. If we only consume food when we are hungry and sleep when we need to then the body knows what to do.

The same is true for feeding the body. The human body was made to store a bit of excess fat in case food is not readily available for a short time. The liver will store up to two days' worth of glycogen that can be turned into ketones when needed for fuel. This is true even in thin people. Early men were hunter-gatherers, meaning they had to hunt for their food and gather those wild fruits and vegetables that they could find. And sometimes food just wasn't available, so the body relied on itself for fuel. But when we began to depend on our modern diets that are full of starches and sugars, then we began to disturb the natural function of the body. Faithfully following the keto lifestyle will reset your internal bodily functions and get your body back to that efficient little machine it always wanted to be.

There are actually several versions of the keto diet that exist and are in use today. Most people use what is known as the standard ketogenic diet. But there is also the cyclical ketogenic diet plan, the targeted ketogenic diet plan, and the high protein keto diet plan.

Those people who are using the cyclical ketogenic diet plan will be allowed to make a choice to rotate the days in which they will have a high consumption of carb intake and other days when they will have low consumption of carb intake. This plan was created to suit a particular style of life. If you are a high functioning athlete or you are training for a marathon then you might well benefit from the cyclical ketogenic diet. This plan also works well for people who have irregular work schedules and do heavy manual labor. This keto plan allows the user to tailor their carb intake to be higher on the days when they will need extra energy, such as days when they work or days when they are training physically. This plan might require a bit more planning than the standard keto diet because you must plan the days when you will eat high carb and the days when you will eat low carb. Since you can't eat high carb every day and lose weight this might take a bit of rearranging until you find the right days to cycle.

The downfall to this plan is that you will still have a steady stream of carbs going into your body so you may never truly adjust to not having carbs as a source of energy. While this is a viable keto plan it might be best to leave this plan until you have been on the standard keto diet for several months. You need to give your body a chance to get used to living without excess starches and sugars and give it a chance to adjust to ketosis.

Many people find that using the targeted keto diet plan is a much more flexible way of doing the keto lifestyle. On this plan, you are allowed to add more carbs into the diet at those times when you will be exercising or otherwise engaging in extra physical activity. Where the cyclical keto diet allows you high carb days when you are physically active, the targeted plan only allows you to eat more carbs within an hour before and an hour after extreme physical activity. This plan is most often used by athletes in training. This plan allows them to take in more carbs just before a period of physical exertion where they will be most likely to burn the carbs as energy during their workout. It also allows them to take in more carbs right after exercising when their metabolisms are still working at peak efficiency and their body will burn the carbs to help in the recovery process. With this plan, it is also recommended that you adhere strictly to the standard keto diet. It is a good idea to adhere to the standard diet for no less than a period of two months and preferably longer in order to allow your body to become fat adapted. This happens when your body has learned to use fat for fuel and will know to quickly burn off the excess carbs and not store them.

The kinds of carbs you eat during the targeted periods are very important also. You will not be allowed to just go wild and eat all the carbs in sight. The idea is to eat the smallest amount possible that will give the effect you are wanting. So it might mean that you are eating a slice or two of bread or a small bowl of rice, but nothing more. And both bread and rice are easily digestible and will turn to sugar quickly in the body.

The high protein ketogenic diet plan is quite similar to the standard keto diet except for the fact that you will consume more protein in this version. The two groups of people that would benefit from this plan the most are older people and those who are devout bodybuilders. The bodybuilders need the added bit of protein in order to grow and maintain good muscle tone and definition. Older people begin to lose muscle mass and they can definitely benefit from the increased protein intake of the high protein keto diet.

If you are following this plan then you will get about one-third of your daily calories from the protein you eat. This may be more difficult to do on the vegetarian keto plan but it can still be done with proper planning.

Those people who have an active kidney disorder are most likely not good candidates for the high protein keto diet plan. Consuming too much protein over an extended period of time could result in a building of waste products in the kidneys and could lead to kidney stones. But if there are no underlying health problems then this keto plan will give the average person the same results and benefits as the standard ketogenic diet plan will.

The most popular plan is called the standard ketogenic diet plan. While using this plan you will consume a low amount of carbs, a moderate amount of proteins, and a high amount of fats. Generally, your diet will be twenty percent protein, seventy-five percent fat, and only five percent carbs. You will determine this by determining what is the overall calorie count of the foods you are consuming in the meal and then dividing those calories into the proper categories.

And while many people say it is not necessary to count calories on the keto diet, even more, people believe that it is. If you are not aware of exactly how many calories you will need to eat every day you will not be able to calculate exactly how many will come from fats, proteins, and carbs. And even if you are eating the right types of foods it is still possible to overeat if you are eating too many calories in total. Whatever you weigh now, there is a calorie amount attached to that number.

It takes _____ calories daily to maintain a body weight of _____ .

If you look online there are any numbers of sites that will tell you exactly how many calories you are consuming daily in order to keep up the weight that you are currently carrying. You do not need to tell anyone what this number is but you do need to know what it is in order to be able to lose weight. For example, if you currently take in three thousand calories a day to maintain your current weight, then you will lose weight if you drop down to two thousand calories or even two thousand five hundred every day. No one ever gained weight overnight and no one will ever lose it overnight. It may be easier to cut out five hundred calories a day and then cut once more when your body adjusts to that.

So besides getting healthier and feeling better, the main goal of the keto diet is to promote weight loss. So how much weight can you realistically hope to lose on the keto diet? A lot of that depends on you personally.

While under normal daily circumstances any person who eats less food will automatically lose weight. It is a simple game of numbers. Your body weight is a direct reflection not only of your lifestyle but also of your genetic makeup. Maybe the people in your family lose weight more slowly. If so then you will probably lose weight more slowly than other people might.

You truly need to know how your body works and to be able to accept the way your body works in order to be able to move on with your weight loss goals. And remember that three thousand five hundred calories make a pound of fat. So cutting three thousand five hundred calories out of your weekly diet will take one pound of weight off of your body every week.

And in the beginning, you will probably lose weight much faster, especially if you are strictly following the keto diet guidelines. This makes sense for several reasons. One reason is that in the beginning, you are losing a lot of water weight. This is because the fat in the body holds water, so as you begin to lose fat the water has nowhere to hide so it must be eliminated through the waste process. So you will find yourself urinating more in the first few weeks. Also, in the first few weeks, you weigh the most you have ever weighed and you are now losing weight, so you will lose more weight quicker in the beginning.

And remember that no one became obese overnight. So after the first few weeks of rapid weight loss losing between one and three pounds weekly is recommended. This gives your body the chance to become used to a much lower intake of calories and to be happy with much less food than before. This slower process is frustrating to many people and they give up before they can really begin to see the results that come from strict adherence to the keto diet.

If you lose two pounds on a regular diet you might be losing water, fat, or muscle; you just never really know. But on the keto diet, after your body has gone through ketosis and is firmly adjusted to the process of burning fat, then two pounds lost is two pounds of fat. And keep in mind that a pound of muscle in the body is smaller than a pound of fat in the body. So your body might start to shrink rapidly even though the scale does not show such a dramatic loss of excess weight. Your body will be shrinking and your clothing will be fitting more loosely.

And different people do lose weight differently. Many people do not consider this when they are beginning a new diet, and then when they don't see the immediate results they expected they give up. Men may naturally lose weight faster than women will because men have higher levels of the hormone testosterone. This hormone makes them manly and helps them to lose weight because they naturally have more muscular bodies and muscle burns more fuel than fat does. And women have high levels of estrogen, the hormone which keeps our bodies ready to feed unborn babies in times of great famine. People who are younger will easily lose weight faster than people who are older because they are younger and more naturally active, and their metabolisms naturally work faster and better than the metabolisms of older people. Someone who is morbidly obese when they begin the keto plan will definitely lose weight faster than most people because they have gone from consuming an enormous amount of calories daily down to consuming a normal amount of calories.

Maintaining the keto diet will require careful planning so that the diet will continue to be successful for you. At first, it may seem to be a lot of extra work to be able to adhere to the keto diet but it is not impossible. The main focus of the diet and the one that will make you successful is finding creative ways to lower your consumption of carbs and keep the level lowered. The majority of people who undertake to live the keto lifestyle will need to consume less than twenty grams of carbs every day. The lower the point you choose to set your carb intake and the better you are at keeping it there the more successful you will be on the keto diet.

Especially in the beginning, it will be important to pay close attention to what you are eating. You should devise a plan to track your food choices and meal plans so that you will know exactly what you are eating in terms of fats, proteins, and carbs. It is never a good idea to guess about your consumption of food. But in the beginning, you need to be sure that your everyday intake of carbs, fats, and proteins stays on the exact ratio you need it to be on. There are many different ways you can choose to do this. Whichever method you decide to use will be the best one for you and your lifestyle. You can create an amazing spreadsheet or download an app from the internet or simply write things down in a spiral notebook. The key is to find the method that works best for you and use it.

The absolute most important thing for you to always remember is that this is a new lifestyle. This is not simply another diet that you will begin and discard when it stops working for you. Keto will work for you for the rest of your life if you do it the right way and allow it to work the way it was meant to work. Take any and all information you can find and use it. Keep searching for new and different recipes to keep your dietary choices interesting. If you are fully prepared to succeed then you definitely will succeed.

Chapter 12: Living Keto In The Real World

Now that you have made the conscious decision to embrace the keto lifestyle you will need to figure out how your life will look when you are out in the world among other people. Because it will be really easy to follow the keto diet strictly when you are at home, even if other people are in your house with you. The trick is when you go out in public. Because even though the keto diet is part of mainstream life right now, and even though more people have heard of the keto way of life than ever before, there will be those people who will question your sanity. After all, you gave up donuts and lattes. Some people will still not believe it is possible to live a perfectly normal life on what they think is a perfectly abnormal style of eating.

But eating low carb is not abnormal. In fact, it was the way our ancestors made it through life so many centuries ago. They ate meat and plants. They did not consume donuts and lattes. But ideas in society evolve very slowly even when solid research is right in front of people. Most people like to believe what they have always believed because they have always believed it.

The problem that is the biggest is that most people have is when they go out to eat with nonketotic living people. On a normal keto style diet is relatively easy to find a good meal at nearly every restaurant because all restaurants serve meat. But when you are living the vegetarian keto lifestyle it might be a bit more restrictive when you are eating out with friends.

There are places in many of the larger cities that cater to a vegan or vegetarian lifestyle. This way of life has become more mainstream in recent years and it is becoming easier to find restaurants whose whole menus are geared toward the eating habits of people who do not consume animals.

If you are going out with friends to any of the family style restaurants, buffet style restaurants, or those with a bar area attached, you should easily be able to find something good to eat. Most of these places feature a large salad bar with an all you can eat option, so you will be busy trying to eat one of every offering on the bar and you definitely will not go hungry. And restaurants that are set up as a one price style buffet pace will not only have a salad bar but will also have a hot vegetable bar so your choices are not limited to cold food.

Dining outside of the house can be a real challenge for vegetarians and vegans. Most restaurants are not necessarily vegan or vegetarian-friendly. Some may have very nice meatless options that they do not tend to advertise or highlight. But by keeping some helpful ideas in mind when eating out you might enjoy a really rewarding experience.

If you are able to then call ahead to the restaurant to see if they offer vegetarian or vegan options. If you know the location where you are going ahead of time this is an easy thing to do. But if this is a spur of the moment group decision you will need to do a bit of extra work. The very first thing that you need to do is to look over the menu to see if you see any dishes that are particularly marked with some symbol that denotes that the dish is vegan or vegetarian. If you don't find any designated dishes or you just don't sure do not be afraid to ask your server. More and more places are training their staff on ways to assist diners with particular food needs.

If you are eating at a fast food place your options might be a bit more limited. Of course, almost every fast-food chain now offers several interesting and flavorful salad options. There are always French fries available on the menu, and many places will serve chili, at least in the colder months. The problem here will be sticking to the keto side of your keto vegetarian diet. A salad just might be your best option. Just ask the staff to make one without the meat.

When you are eating at a friend's house it is perfectly acceptable to ask what is being served and to reiterate that you are a vegetarian. Your real friends will already know this and will have options available for you, or they might suggest that you bring something with you.

When you are traveling it is usually easy to get the kind of food that you need to be eating. Trains, airlines, and especially cruise ships are becoming increasingly aware of and trying to cater to the dietary needs of a wider group of people. After all, people using their services are how they make their money. So it is definitely in their best interests to work to be able to meet the nutritional needs of as many people as possible.

Those restaurants that are considered global cuisine might be the best option for locating vegetarian food. Those places that feature a decided Asian theme, like Vietnamese, Thai, Japanese, and Chinese will have menus that will feature a good variety of menu options that have no meat and this will include noodle dishes and rice dishes that contain tofu and vegetables. Be sure to ask your server if the dish will contain oyster or fish sauce. Those places that feature a more South Asian cuisine like Nepalese, Pakistani, Burmese, Sri Lankan, and Indian are well known for serving dishes without meat that feature yogurts, curried vegetables, rice, beans, lentils, and bread. Dishes will be prepared using oil or butter so you will be able to maintain your fat intake for the day.

Restaurants that serve Middle Eastern, Greek, Italian, And Mediterranean foods will definitely have an abundance of meatless menu options. Here you will find tabbouleh, Greek salads, dishes made with eggplant, minestrone and other vegetable-based soups, couscous, falafel, pasta marinara, and pasta primavera. Especially in the Mediterranean locations, your food will be prepared using large amounts of oil so this will help with your fat intake.

Mexican cuisine is usually quite vegetarian-friendly. With options like tamales, quesadillas, enchiladas, tacos, fajitas, and burritos made with cheese, beans, and rice there should be something available for any vegetarian to eat. Salsa, guacamole, and Spanish rice are definitely vegetarian options, as are refried beans.

Certain food items are almost guaranteed to be vegetarian and can be found at many restaurants. Look for soups and stir-fries, as these are often one hundred percent vegetarian. Look for choices that include tempeh, edamame, and tofu to guarantee a good source of protein.

Just remember that your dietary choices are yours. Most restaurants will assist the diner in getting an option that fits their dietary needs. If you do not see a specific vegetarian option on a menu then ask the server. Often times you can mix items from two different menu options to come up with a viable vegetarian option. And always be sure to reiterate that you will eat no meat, chicken, or fish. People do not always think of fish or chicken as being left out of a vegetarian diet; they usually just think of beef.

When eating out as you may have noticed some of the suggestions are definitely vegetarian and at the same time definitely not keto friendly. Unfortunately, when eating out you may not be able to keep vegetarian and keep keto. Obviously, vegetarianism is a lifestyle that you chose for a reason so does not feel the least bit bad about choosing to stay vegetarian even if your choices are not in line with the keto diet. One meal of carbs will not be enough to derail your progress or knock you out of ketosis. Just do not make a regular habit of eating out in places that do not offer keto options that are vegetarian and you will be just fine.

Just remember that dining out is not a way of life and keto is. But there will be times when you just can't or do not want to avoid eating out in public with other people. At these times it is important to just do your best, and if you need to fall off the keto wagon for one meal then just get back on at your first opportunity. Because you are doing this so that your life can be more enjoyable overall, and that is what life is all about.

Conclusion

Thank you for making it through to the end of Keto Vegetarian Diet: The Ultimate Guide to the Ketogenic Vegetarian Diet for Permanent Weight Loss and Burn Fat; Includes Easy Low-Carb Plant-Based Recipes, Beginner Friendly by Michelle Thomasson, let's hope it was informative and able to provide you with a complete set of the tools you need to achieve your goals whatever they may be.

The next step is to use what you have learned in this book to take charge of your life and your weight loss goals and begin your journey on the path to your new lifestyle. You have already made the lifestyle decision to eat vegetarian foods, now add to that decision the choice to eat a keto lifestyle. By adding these two lifestyle choices together you will have the two most powerful weapons for weight loss and healthy living at your disposal. You now possess all the knowledge that you need in order to make this new lifestyle change to keto vegetarianism.

The different herbs and spices that were featured in this book have shown you how easy it is to create tasty dishes. You have recipes for many different sauces that will help to compliment your vegetarian choices without totally blowing your keto diet plan. You have recipes for delicious breakfasts, lunches, and dinners. We showed you how to create a sample meal plan that will teach you how easy it is to make good choices when it comes to the food that you put in your body. And we even gave you some recipes for desserts because we know you are human and life is so much better when it includes a little treat every now and then.

Most importantly we hope you now see that living the keto vegetarian lifestyle is not impossible. It might not be one of the easiest things you will ever do but it will enrich your life and your health far beyond anything you might ever have imagined.

Finally, if you found this book useful in any way, a review on Amazon is always appreciated!

Printed in Great Britain
by Amazon